KNOWLEDGE TO ACTI

Knowledge to Action?

Evidence-Based Health Care in Context

Edited by
SUE DOPSON
and
LOUISE FITZGERALD

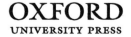

OXFORD
UNIVERSITY PRESS

OXFORD
UNIVERSITY PRESS

Great Clarendon Street, Oxford OX2 6DP

Oxford University Press is a department of the University of Oxford.
It furthers the University's objective of excellence in research, scholarship,
and education by publishing worldwide in

Oxford New York

Auckland Cape Town Dar es Salaam Hong Kong Karachi
Kuala Lumpur Madrid Melbourne Mexico City Nairobi
New Delhi Shanghai Taipei Toronto

With offices in

Argentina Austria Brazil Chile Czech Republic France Greece
Guatemala Hungary Italy Japan Poland Portugal Singapore
South Korea Switzerland Thailand Turkey Ukraine Vietnam

Oxford is a registered trade mark of Oxford University Press
in the UK and in certain other countries

Published in the United States
by Oxford University Press Inc., New York

British Library Cataloguing in Publication Data

Data available

Library of Congress Cataloging in Publication Data

Knowledge to action? : evidence based health care in context/
edited by Sue Dopson and Louise Fitzgerald.
p. cm.
Includes bibliographical references and index.
1. Evidence-based medicine–Great Britain. I. Dopson, Sue.
II. Fitzgerald, Louise, 1945-
R723.7.K66 2005   616–dc22   2005001533

Typeset by SPI Publisher Services, Pondicherry, India
Printed in Great Britain
on acid-free paper by
Biddles Ltd., King's Lynn, Norfolk

ISBN 0-19-925901-1   978-0-19-925901-4
ISBN 0-19-920510-8 (Pbk.)   978-0-19-920510-3 (Pbk.)

1 3 5 7 9 10 8 6 4 2

For Julian and William
Sue

For Tim, Louise, and Ellie
Louise F

For Tom and Joyce Ferlie
Ewan

For Steve, Alex, and Freddie
Louise L

Acknowledgements

We acknowledge those organizations and individuals whose interest, support, and encouragement have enabled us to write this book:

Dame Sandra Dawson
Kim Sutherland
Rachel Miller
David Chambers
Susan Law
Rebecca Surrender
Martin Wood

Contents

Contents

List of Tables

List of Figures

List of Appendices

Abbreviations

AHP	Allied health professionals
ARIF	Aggressive Research Intelligence Facility
CHC	Community Health Council
CPD	Continuous professional development
CSAG	Clinical Standards Advisory Group
CTG	Cardiotocogram
D&C	Dilation and curettage
DoH	Department of Health
EBHC	Evidence-based health care
EBM	Evidence-based medicine
EBP	Evidence-based policy
ENT	Ear, nose, and throat
EPOC	Effective Practice and Organization of Care
ESRC	Economic and Social Research Council
GP	General practitioner
GRiPP	Getting Research into Practice and Purchasing
HA	Health Authority
HEFCE	Higher Education Funding Council for England
HSR	Health Services Research
LMWH	Low-molecular-weight heparin
NHS	National Health Service
NHSCRD	National Health Service Centre for Reviews and Dissemination
NICE	National Institute of Clinical Excellence
NPM	New public management
NRAF	Non-rheumatic atrial fibrillation
NSF	National Service Framework
OB	Organizational behaviour
PACE	Promoting Action on Clinical Effectiveness
RCT	Randomized control trial
R&D	Research and development
RHA	Regional Health Authority
RRTP	Relating research to practice
TQM	Total quality management
UKCC	United Kingdom Central Council for Nursing, Midwifery and Health Visiting

1

Introduction

Sue Dopson and Louise Fitzgerald

Health services can and should be improved by applying research findings about good practice. This book describes why it is, nevertheless, so notoriously difficult to implement research evidence in the face of strong professional views and complex organizational contexts. It is an empirical study, grounded in the experiences of those dealing with innovation processes in health care.

The issue of how to diffuse and implement innovations has become a burgeoning area of research in many organizations, including health care settings. In the UK, it is an important topic within the health care policy context. Planned improvements in the quality and delivery of health care, it is argued, will only be obtainable if new knowledge is used in relevant and appropriate ways within the health service. The prominence of these issues is also directly related to the push to apply the principles of evidence-based health care (EBHC) within clinical practice. The EBHC movement centres on the results of a great deal of research that suggest a significant gap between what information is available and what is done in clinical practice. It advocates ensuring that clinical practice is continually informed by the results of 'robust' research. For the past several years, EBHC has been viewed by many policy-makers, managers, and clinicians as an important lever to ensure clinical practice is more effective and represents value for money.

In this book we are specifically interested in what we regard to be under-researched questions concerning the latter stages of the creation, diffusion, and adoption of new knowledge, namely: What makes this information credible and therefore utilized? Why do actors decide to use new knowledge? What is the significance of the social context of which actors are a part? The book also attempts to address these questions in a novel way, in that it arises from regular meetings of two groups of researchers working within the rapidly developing field of health services research (HSR) in the UK, which have over the last four years sought to reflect on their activity and knowledge of research in relation to these questions. In particular, we have considered whether it would be additive to 'scale up' or aggregate analyses by taking an overview across a suite of seven related and recently completed studies that consider the diffusion of innovation. Findings from these seven studies have been brought together in this book, comprising forty-nine separate case studies. More than 1,400 interviews were carried out across the studies. Further details on the background to each piece of research and the team involved in each are provided in Appendix 1.1. This appendix is important as it documents the nature of the studies we were involved in and the source of our tacit knowledge that we have brought to bear on the analysis of these issues.

The team members involved in the work presented in this book come from a variety of disciplinary backgrounds, including organizational behaviour (OB) and management, sociology, social policy, and public health, but all with a particular research focus on health care organization and management. At the time the original research was carried out, one research team was based at Warwick University, Centre for Corporate Strategy and Change, and the other had members based at both Templeton College, Oxford and Wessex Institute for Health Research & Development, University of Southampton. One of the studies also involved the Judge Institute of Management Studies, University of Cambridge, and another involved the Department of Social Policy and Social Work, University of Oxford.

We were interested in exploring, firstly, if 'pooling' results across this family of related studies would produce more generalizable findings in relation to attempts to introduce the principles of EBHC into the National Health Service (NHS) and, secondly, if so, what are the rules of method to be adopted and do they differ from those apparent within the conventional systematic review paradigm? We were also keen to make an analytical contribution to the existing literature on innovation studies, as well as to explore possible policy implications.

1.1   The organization of the book

Following this brief introduction are seven chapters. Chapter 2 reviews the field of organizational studies as a whole in order to provide a background to the arguments raised in subsequent chapters. The proposition is advanced that EBHC is likely to be imperfectly implemented through uniform approaches within such highly complex and variable settings characteristic of health care. This suggests the need for finely grained and holistic analyses of the processes of implementation within 'real life' clinical settings.

Chapter 3 considers the origins and rise of EBHC and explores some of the reactions to it, notably amongst doctors themselves, managers, and policy-makers. The 'implementation gap' between what is planned and what is actually achieved is explored by drawing on existing studies. This chapter provides an important backdrop to the detailed presentation of our attempt to upscale our qualitative work in this area. Chapter 4 contains details of our empirical study, and how we worked together on our upscaling project. It also considers more generally the State of HSR and the signs of rigour within qualitative research.

Chapters 5, 6, 7, and 8 comprise the key themes that emerged from our collective review of the empirical data available to us from the studies. These include the active role of context in the translation of evidence into clinical practice (Chapter 5); the influence of the distinctive nature of professionalized organization (Chapter 6); the contested nature of evidence (Chapter 7); and the complex ways in which evidence becomes potentially applicable to local practice before it becomes actionable knowledge (Chapter 8). Knowledge in action for us is therefore evidence that has been converted through social processes into locally accepted knowledge, which is then put into use and leads to evidence-based change in working practice.

The concluding chapter reviews the key themes and spells out what we hope you will consider to be a contribution to existing debates.

Appendix 1.1   Descriptions of the Seven Studies

This appendix contains a brief description of the background to, and content of, each study. The references given are for the final report of each study. The members of each separate research team are listed. Members of the joint team involved in developing an overview of all the studies are highlighted in bold.

GRiPP (Getting Research into Practice and Purchasing)

GRiPP (Dopson and Gabbay 1995) was the first study, commissioned by the then Anglia and Oxford Regional Health Authority (RHA). The GRiPP initiative started in 1993, with £100,000 funding from the National Health Service Management Executive (NHSME), and was intended to explore ways in which research evidence could be used to inform health care purchasing decisions. Each of the four counties in the region selected a clinical topic: surgery for children with suspected glue-ear; better coordinated care for stroke patients; the use of corticosteroids for women expected to deliver prematurely; and elective dilatation and curettage (D&C) in women under forty. Each project assembled available evidence and sought to involve local clinicians and managers in deciding what should be done on the basis of the evidence and then implementing change. The evaluation of the project was commissioned to help participants learn from the process and develop recommendations for the conduct of similar initiatives in the future.

GRiPP team

Sue Dopson, Oxford   **John Gabbay**, Southampton

PACE (Promoting Action on Clinical Effectiveness)

GRiPP exercised a direct influence on a subsequent initiative, PACE (Dopson et al. 1999). Mike Dunning, originally seconded from the

Department of Health (DoH) to Anglia and Oxford for the GRiPP initiative, moved to the King's Fund in London to run a nationwide demonstration project funded by the DoH, to develop further the work carried out under the GRiPP initiative. PACE ran for two years from 1997 and involved sixteen projects, two in each of the eight regions of the NHS. PACE topic areas were hypertension, *Helicobacter pylori* (three sites), pressure sores, menorrhagia, continence (two sites), stroke, congestive cardiac failure, post-operative pain control, leg ulcers, stable angina, low back pain, and family support in schizophrenia. The DoH commissioned the same team to evaluate PACE and identify emerging lessons.

PACE team

Sue Dopson, Oxford   **John Gabbay**, Southampton
Sue Law, Oxford (first year)   **Louise Locock**, Oxford (second year)
David Chambers,
Oxford (second year)

Warwick Acute Study

The first of the two Warwick studies (Wood et al. 1998) was commissioned by the Organisation and Management Group of the North Thames NHS Regional Research and Development (R&D) Directorate for two years from 1995. Unlike GRiPP and PACE, this was not an evaluation of a specially constituted demonstration project, but aimed rather at exploring the implementation of effectiveness evidence within normal working practices. Four clinical topic areas were selected; the aim was to examine two areas in both medicine and surgery where the research evidence seemed to be strongly supportive of change and to command consensus (oral anticoagulation therapy and thromboprophylaxis in orthopaedic surgery respectively) and two where the evidence was more ambivalent or contested (changing childbirth and laparoscopic surgery for inguinal hernia repair). One case study was conducted for each topic area.

Warwick Acute Study team

Martin Wood, Warwick   **Ewan Ferlie**, Warwick
Louise Fitzgerald, Warwick

RRTP (Relating Research to Practice)

RRTP (Dawson et al. 1998) was also commissioned by the Organisation and Management Group of the North Thames NHS Regional R&D Directorate for two years from 1995. Again, this was a study of the implementation of effectiveness evidence in normal organizational settings, not an evaluation of a demonstration project. The research focused on the management of asthma in adults and glue ear in children. A total of four case studies were carried out, two for each clinical topic. Each involved an acute hospital setting and a sample of surrounding general practitioners (GPs). Two hospitals were in North Thames Region and two in Anglia and Oxford Region.

RRTP team

Sandra Dawson, Cambridge

Sue Dopson, Oxford

Sue Law, Oxford

Kim Sutherland, Cambridge

Rachel Miller, Cambridge

CSAG (Clinical Standards Advisory Group)

CSAG was established in 1991 as an independent source of expert advice to ministers and the NHS on clinical standards in the NHS. The Health Departments (England, Wales, and Scotland) commissioned CSAG to investigate the impact of clinical effectiveness evidence on services for patients during 1996–7. A total of thirteen case studies were carried out on one clinical topic (the management of patients with stroke) (CSAG 1998).

CSAG team

John Gabbay

John Acres

Leigh Appleby

Ann Ashburn

Sally Bailey

Jane Dawson

Lynn Kerridge

(All researchers from Southampton)

James Raftery

Paul Roderick

Amanda Samuel

Martin Severs

Kenneth Stein

Eileen Thomas

Daniel Warm

Warwick Primary Care Study

The Warwick Primary Care Study (Fitzgerald et al. 1999) was commissioned for two years from 1997, and was funded by the West Midlands Region R&D Directorate. It was designed to develop and complement the work done for the acute study and compare findings in the less well-researched setting of primary care. Similar methods were therefore used. Four case studies were carried out, one on each of four clinical topic areas. The Warwick Primary Care Study clinical topics were use of aspirin for prevention of secondary cardiac incidents, treatment of diabetes in primary care following the St Vincent declaration, use of hormone replacement therapy for treatment of osteoporosis, and employment of physiotherapists in primary care.

Warwick Primary Care Study team

Louise Fitzgerald, De Montfort   **Ewan Ferlie**, Imperial College
Chris Hawkins, Warwick

Welsh Clinical Effectiveness Initiative National Demonstration Projects

The former Welsh Office established six demonstration projects in Wales to test out the implementation of clinical effectiveness evidence in five clinical topic areas. Welsh Demonstration Project topics were stroke (two sites), schizophrenia, pressure sores, diabetes, and emergency hospital admissions. The Welsh Office commissioned the Oxford/Southampton team to evaluate the demonstration projects, with particular emphasis on gathering qualitative data about participants' experience (Locock et al. 1999). The evaluation, which took place during 1998–9, developed the methodology used in the PACE evaluation.

Welsh Project team

Louise Locock, Oxford   **John Gabbay**, Southampton
Sue Dopson, Oxford   Rebecca Surender, Oxford
David Chambers, Oxford

2

Studying Complex Organizations in Health Care

Ewan Ferlie and Sue Dopson

2.1 Introduction

The majority of statements from policy-makers and in policy documents on evidence-based health care (EBHC) implementation draw
on classic diffusion of innovation models, the most influential of
which remains Rogers' (1995). Rogers argues that the adoption of
new ideas, practices, and artefacts is influenced by the interaction
among the innovation, the adopter, and the environment. In his view
there are five characteristics that influence the success rate of adoption: the perception of the relative advantage of innovation; the com-
patibility with existing structures; the degree of difficulty involved in
making the change; the extent to which the innovation can be tested
by potential adopters without significant resource expenditure; and
the visibility of the outcomes. Rogers' early work has been criticized
for adopting a rational view of how change is achieved and for its
simplicity in relation to the complexity of the change process. Furthermore, while his later work (from 1995) explicitly considers the
nature of the adoption process within large organizations rather than
by individuals, a unitary perspective is still evident; for example,
according to Rogers, later stages in the innovation process cannot be
undertaken until earlier stages have been settled, either explicitly or
implicitly.

Rational models of the innovation process have been challenged
within the general literature on innovation. A selection of this work is
given below to illustrate the emerging themes. Williams and Gibson
(1990) suggest a sequence of four models of diffusion: the *appropriability model* (science push); *dissemination model* (good science, plus
strong networks and communications, boundary spanners); *knowledge utilization model* (incorporating demand pull, problem-solving

needs among the users); and the *communication and feedback model*. These authors describe the innovation process as being dependent on communication between stakeholders, where researchers, developers, and users may have differing perspectives about the innovation, which must be accommodated for diffusion to occur. In short, they see the dissemination process as far more chaotic than the S-curve used in Rogers' work suggests. While their model acknowledges the importance of feedback loops, it does not, however, provide an analysis of the complex social context that is often referred to in the literature as the 'receiving system'.

Kimberly (1981) argues that the existing literature concentrates on the adoption behaviour of individuals and neglects the fact that the career of managerial innovations is shaped in particular by the internal change capacity of the receiving organization and the context in which it is situated. He points out that while environmental constraints are often acknowledged conceptually, they have rarely been examined empirically. The relationship between organizational attributes and innovation has been explored by Damanpour (1991), who provides a list of independent organizational variables and their expected relationship to innovation.

Argyris and Schon (1996) have argued that the diffusion process is frequently decentralized and iterative in nature and that a key aspect of the diffusion of innovation is the capacity of the organization to learn about the context of their learning. Actor network theory (Latour 1987) and the emerging literature on the importance of communities of practice (discussed in more detail below) point to social networks and communities of knowledge as critical to gaining scientific acceptance for ideas. They are considered important features of the innovation process that need to receive much more attention from researchers.

A 'community of practice' (Wenger 1998: 45) has been seen as a work-related community created through the sustained collective pursuit of a shared enterprise. It provides a strong basis for collective learning and change. Single professional-based groups and associated networks provide an authentic and powerful community of practice in that they provide a prime basis for face-to-face interaction, information and experience exchange, and learning activity in relation to day-to-day health care practices—but usually for members of the same profession. Interactions within such a community of practice are said to be 'richer' than with higher managerial tiers of the organization or other communities of practice. The professional communities of practice we encountered display features that differ from the non-professional work contexts analysed by Wenger. Firstly, professional communities of practice are often unidisciplinary in nature, and great effort is needed to create a functioning multidisciplinary community of practice. Secondly, they typically seal themselves off, even (or perhaps especially) from neighbouring professional communities of practice, defending jurisdictions and group identity.

Brown and Duguid (2001*a*) examine the way knowledge manifests 'stickiness' and 'leakiness' simultaneously. They argue that sociocultural accounts offer richer explanations than focusing on the properties of knowledge itself. By shifting their analysis to concrete practice, they underline the link between learning and identity, arguing that work identities are built through participation and social contact. Knowledge diffuses within communities of practice, but it will stick where practice is not shared. As argued earlier, the presence of strong professional roles and identities makes it even less likely that knowledge will flow across social boundaries.

Jelinek and Schoonhoven's work (1990) on innovation in high technology firms also suggests the value of paying more attention to interconnections, multiple teams, multiple relationships, and interactions. Finally we have ourselves stressed that local actors—and the interactions between these actors—are a major source of the messy and unpredictable nature of the innovation process empirically apparent within health care (Ferlie et al. 2001). Emergent change was found to be far more evident than planned change, and innovations have to be enacted within local clinical groups that are well able to resist change initiatives.

This developing literature challenges the sequential view of the career of the innovation and stresses its messy, dynamic, and fluid nature. It has informed the literature of EBHC implementation, acknowledging the need for multiple models to explain such a complex social process. Despite such developments, a great deal of the text aims at assisting those charged with achieving evidence-based change locally to fall back on more linear models, where knowledge and implementation are viewed as relatively unproblematic. Unfortunately in the UK, it is often such texts that are seized upon by policy-makers in their deliberations in this area. Such linear accounts falsely imply that the many stakeholders within health care organizations are united in a common purpose to promote the use of EBHC and that, furthermore, the evidence presented in relation to clinical practice is often conclusive. Both these assumptions should be questioned.

In this chapter we argue instead that health care organizations are themselves far from unitary in character, displaying a range of different professions and other interest groups, each with their own agendas to advance and 'jurisdictions' to protect. The available evidence in favour of an innovation is often partial and ambiguous. Different health care professions respond to and produce different forms of evidence. Evidence has to be interpreted and 'enacted' within particular work settings, which are dependent on negotiation and agreement with other stakeholders. This chapter considers how we should analyse these organizational settings and how their characteristics add complexity and variability to the enactment of EBHC in clinical practice.

2.2   Key research traditions within organizational studies

Organizational studies is a developing social science with links to sociological forms of analysis. Organizational studies in the UK emerged in the 1950s and 1960s, initially with a focus on how underlying technology was related to the organization of work (Woodward 1965). Key elements of work structure could be identified and measured, often using structured scaling techniques. Many of the underlying assumptions were functionalist (certain forms of organizational structure sprang from a technological base or other external drivers and represented an efficient fit) and positivistic (underlying dimensions of organizational structure were capable of measurement). The studies of the so-called Aston Group were particularly influential, developing a 'contingency theoretic' approach to the study and measurement of key dimensions of organizational structure, which was found to vary with external factors (Pugh 1997).

This original tradition still has its adherents, who see it as a way of building a 'normal' management science (Donaldson 1996). It is hoped that repeatable studies can provide evidence about fundamental organizational 'laws'. This tradition remains strong in American management studies. However, the dominant position of structural contingency theory within organizational studies in the UK rapidly eroded in the 1980s (Whitley 2000), and a myriad of competing specialisms and conceptual approaches took its place. The overall trend (Clegg et al. 1996) has been from formal to more informal accounts of organization. Under this broad umbrella, there has been a proliferation of new and different approaches, essentially mirroring similar developments in neighbouring social sciences such as sociology or social policy. This 'mega shift' led to a move away from the use of quantitative methods (such as scaling and modelling) associated with structural contingency theory towards less traditional methods. By contrast, there is today not one organizational theory or perspective but many. There is a proliferation of emerging feminist, neo-Marxist, and postmodernist groupings alongside more orthodox groupings of quantitative and indeed qualitative researchers (who themselves can be seen as methodologically more conservative than some of the newer groupings).

Reflecting on recent shifts in organizational analysis a number of significant changes have occurred. Firstly there has been a move away from grand theory to generating theory from empirical work, known as grounded theory (Glaser and Strauss 1967). Secondly, scholars have sought to study issues of power, culture, and theory, rather than seeking to study and control how organizations are ordered. Finally, scholars have moved from the study of situational contingencies and environmental determinism to how the study of strategic choice is exercised (Child 1972, 1997; Child and Smith 1987) and how actors construct their environment via the process of enactment (Weick 1969, 1995).

2.3   Qualitative organizational research

Qualitative organizational research represents a counter-orientation to structuralist and quantitative approaches. It has a long international history that predates the early UK studies of the 1950s and 1960s already alluded to. It has strong sociological roots going back to the great founder of organizational sociology—Max Weber—and his emphasis on *verstehen* within social research (Weber 1978, 1990), which is the interpretive understanding of the meaning that humans attach to their actions. While the American management research culture is today mainly positivistic, this may be regarded as somewhat odd because American academics have also produced highly significant qualitative social and organizational research. From the 1930s to 1960s, the so-called Chicago School of urban sociology in particular produced a succession of classic texts that explored the day-to-day experience of marginal or deviant subgroups within organizations, often using intensive observation and other qualitative methods. This included accounts of a mental hospital as seen from the patients' perspective (Goffman 1963) or of a Medical School as seen by the students (Becker et al. 1961). Alternative methodological perspectives to quantitative analysis were strongly evident, notably the use of ethnography (Goffman 1963), whereby a researcher became deeply immersed in an organization in order to identify its day-to-day working practices and to understand how it 'really' operated. Espoused or 'front stage' accounts of organizational purpose could vary markedly from the behaved or 'back stage' reality uncovered through ethnography.

2.4   Three core models of organization

Here we draw on the work of Hatch (1997), who usefully distinguishes between three overall perspectives on organizations that are currently evident—the modernist, the symbolic interpretive, and the post-modernist.

2.4.1   *Modernist perspective*

Hatch (1997: 34–41) argues that the modernist perspective on organizations essentially sees them as systems. The organizational system can be divided into different subsystems (e.g. a company may have specialist Marketing and Research Departments), but these in turn are integrated by linking mechanisms, such as joint teams. The organizational system is located within the 'supersystem' of the environment to which it relates. Moreover, there is a hierarchy of systems that generates 'levels' of work (such as top management, middle management, and supervisors), all of which operate differently. In modernist organization theory, roles can be defined differently according to their level in the formal hierarchy. So top management's perspective is usually conceptualized in terms of the organization's relationship with the environment, and operates at the highest or strategic level. Middle management relates to the internal activities of the organization, and is especially concerned with translating top management's strategic vision into operational action. The perspective of a 'supervisor' is equated with the day-to-day problems of managing a small group of workers (Hatch 1997: 40). The modernist perspective analyses organizations in formal and structural terms.

Methodologically, the modernist perspective is aligned to structural contingency theory and to positivistic methods, which use statistical measurement techniques (such as formal scaling or multi-variate statistical analyses) in order to produce comparative quantitative studies of formal organizational structures. The well-known work of the Aston Group on plotting and predicting where organizations would lie on formally measured dimensions of organizing (such as centralization or formalization) would be a good example of such an approach (Pugh 1981, 1997).

2.4.2 *Symbolic interpretive perspective, enactment, and the social construction of reality*

Hatch (1997) considers the symbolic interpretive perspective within organizational studies particularly associated with the work of Weick (1969) (although, as has been mentioned, Weber and the Chicago School sociologists are important earlier influences). The informal organization is here seen as more important than the formal organization, which may exist solely on an organization chart. 'Real' organizational life is constructed or 'enacted' in Weickian terms within particular work settings. A clinical team would be a good example of such enactment of a negotiated order, in which participants learn to work with each other through repeated interpersonal encounters around joint tasks. Of course, some participants (such as consultants within medical teams) have a higher degree of power than other team members, and are able to influence the ways in which work roles are enacted.

Weick's enactment theory focuses on the subjective rather than objective origin of organizational 'realities'. An organization is enacted by people developing particular work practices, rather than existing objectively and independently of social action. For example, modernist contingency theory assumes that the 'environment' determines the nature of the organization. However, symbolic interpretivist scholars would argue that such environmental forces have to be sensed and analysed by organizational decision-makers. Such decision-makers use their interpretations of the environment to take actions they deem appropriate—in a sense they create the environment to which they then respond. Some managerial teams may be much better at sensing environmental changes than others. So organizational orders are negotiated by social actors, consistent with a view that reality is socially constructed (Berger and Luckman 1966). Subjective factors such as values, beliefs, culture, and language all emerge as important concepts that help explain how these negotiated orders are held together. The symbolic interpretive perspective is aligned with the use of such methods as participant observation, organizational ethnographies, and intensive case studies. This allows for the intensive observation of micro decision-making groups, such as senior management teams or indeed clinical teams. We would locate ourselves broadly within this tradition.

2.4.3 *Postmodern organizational theory*

Hatch (1997) sees postmodernist ideas in organizational theory as evolving out of the post-structuralist movement in French philosophy of the 1970s. It found its way into organization theory through applications of linguistic and literary theory. It developed in opposition to modernism and its search for 'grand narratives' or (within organization theory) general predictive models. The fragmentation and extreme diversity of current societies and work roles is a favourite theme. Postmodern frames of analysis are seen to fit well with post-industrial societies, where people work in small, more decentralized, informal, and flexible organizations. Postmodernists also dispute traditional theories of scientific knowledge, arguing that intuition or aesthetic experience may be equally valid ways of knowing as traditional forms of science. Modernist theory is seen not as a science but as an ideological legitimation of the power held by managerial elites. Postmodernists critique the power held by managerial elites, seeking to reclaim the silence of marginalized elements within organizations (such as women or ethnic minorities) by giving them a voice. So all accounts should be 'deconstructed' to see who they benefit, and in order to escape from totalizing accounts that seek one right solution. The postmodern approach demands a considerable degree of self-reflexivity, a willingness to engage in a voyage of self-exploration and to overturn taken-for-granted assumptions about organizational life.

Methodologically, the postmodernist model is aligned with novel methods such as deconstruction, pastiche, collage, the use of metaphors as a way of understanding organizations, and the critique of theorizing practices. There is a production of highly reflexive accounts, which seek to expose the interests and motivations of the authors. This approach tends to be highly critical of the modernist stance of science and technology and their research traditions.

2.5   Organizational studies and the analysis of health care organizations: differing development patterns

We now move on from an overview of the field of organizational studies as a whole to consider more specific ways in which researchers have examined health care organizations (the contribution of the separate health services research [HSR] stream of literature will be considered later). Well-conducted qualitative organizational analyses using a broadly symbolic interpretive perspective were pioneered in health care organizations by the Chicago School (Becker et al. 1961; Goffman 1963). The quantitative analysis of health care organizations remains a strong tradition, especially in the USA, where quantitative approaches have superseded the Chicago School legacy. For example, a well-conducted study by Budetti et al. (2000) examined the relationship between the implementation of total quality management (TQM) programmes within health care organizations, organizational culture, and final clinical outcomes for a group of coronary artery bypass surgery patients. Interestingly, it attempted to explore the relationship between intermediate process indicators and final clinical outcomes. Quantitative data on TQM implementation and organizational culture were gathered by structured instruments and then subjected to modelling techniques. In the end it was found that the presence of TQM programmes and a supportive organizational culture were not significantly associated with differences in many quality and clinical outcome variables.

Turning from US to UK literature on health care organizations, current academic work appears more dominated by qualitative methods and a symbolic interpretive perspective than apparent in the USA. This pattern is found also in other branches of UK public management research. Boyne (2001) plaintively comments that the quantitative tradition in UK public management research that appeared to be establishing itself in the 1960s and 1970s has, if anything, disappeared (this appears to be the reverse pattern to the American experience). Ferlie's review (2002) of the State of UK health care management research identified a pattern. The published articles examined in two key management journals sympathetic to public management were found to be overwhelmingly drawn from an organizational behaviour (OB) perspective rather than from other important subdisciplines within management, such as marketing or strategy. These OB-based studies usually used qualitative and interpretive methods, especially case studies. There were very few articles found using either a modernist perspective or a postmodern perspective. Symbolic interpretive methods were dominant and could now be seen as the tradition of 'normal science' established in this field.

However, there were significant weaknesses found in these articles, which need to be considered. Firstly, there was a strong tradition in these articles to emerge from the results of policy-based and applied evaluations. There was an overconnection to a research agenda set by the policy domain and a consequent failure to access and develop social science theory (some would argue that this is simply another example of the applied and policy-driven nature of much social science in the UK). Secondly, many of the studies were extremely small-scale, and while they may have had strong internal validity (i.e. they presented insightful and rich accounts of the organizations studied), they were low on external validity such that one would hesitate to generalize from the small sample to the population of organizations. While we will also use case study methods, this book seeks to make two contributions to this pre-existing stream of literature. Firstly, we will 'pool' a set of case-study-based research and our collective knowledge of research in this area, which, taken as a whole, will display a higher degree of external validity than found in conventional case-study-based research. We have had the benefit of working in research teams—rather than on an individual basis—which allowed for an unusual scope within fieldwork design. Secondly, while the studies on which we drew originally were indeed commissioned as applied and policy-relevant evaluations, we now seek to move beyond applied analysis towards a more sustained application and development of social science theory in relation to EBHC implementation.

2.6   The current literature on EBHC implementation and an organizational 'gap'

We now move to consider some more specific questions: What do we already know about EBHC implementation? Where are the gaps or controversies in the present stock of knowledge? Are there methodological controversies apparent in this field? We start by acknowledging that EBHC implementation is an area of interest to both the clinical and social sciences. Biomedical and organizational approaches to the study of EBHC implementation have diverged, at least in the UK. This is unsurprising as they reflect different research 'paradigms' or assumptions about what constitutes high-quality knowledge. Oakley (2001) gives an interesting account of the differences between positivistic and interpretive research paradigms in HSR.

It has been empirically concluded that projects designed to implement research evidence within clinical practice have taken much longer than originally intended (Evans and Haines 2000): it is common ground that there is an implementation gap (discussed in more detail in Chapter 3). How do we respond to this important empirical conclusion? The two research traditions propose different agendas in response to this finding. Researchers influenced by the biomedical tradition are primarily concerned with the development of a science of EBHC guideline implementation (Gross and Romano 2001). This work has been strongly influenced by a Cochrane-based model stressing the importance of systematic reviews of rigorous studies, especially randomized control trials (RCTs), as the highest form of evidence. While there is an awareness that context matters, there is still a preference for the development of RCT-based forms of knowledge. As Bero et al. (1998) argue:

[D]isentangling the effects of intervention from the influence of contextual factors is difficult when interpreting the results of individual trials of behavioural change. Nevertheless, systematic reviews of rigorous studies provide the best evidence of the effectiveness of different strategies for effecting behavioural change.

Grimshaw et al. (2001) made a useful overview of systematic reviews of interventions designed to translate EBHC-related research into practice. Their focus was to identify interventions where there was good quality evidence of broad effectiveness, that is across different health care settings, systems and time periods. Their survey included previous studies that had used a variety of methods, which they sought to weigh according to quality criteria. They stressed the need to develop more rigorous evaluation, which would include more experimental and quasi-experimental designs (Grimshaw et al. 2000) as a priority. They concluded that, in general, passive approaches to implementing EBHC are ineffective. Most other interventions are effective in some circumstances: none are effective in all circumstances (as contextual forms of analysis would indeed argue). Promising approaches include educational outreach (for prescribing) and reminders. Multifaceted interventions targeted to change different barriers are more likely to be effective than single interventions.

By way of comment, we argue that this work suggests that there are important 'effect modifiers' (to use terms appropriate to the methodology used) that inhibit the development of evidence about the general laws, which were perhaps originally hoped for. There may indeed be more modifiers than effects, which means that it is difficult to isolate strong effects. These reviews suggest that the effectiveness of interventions may indeed vary strongly by context. Where there is evidence of strong and consistent effects across studies, it is often confined to particular sectors (such as prescribing) from which it is difficult to generalize. These approaches can be seen as dominated by the search for empirical mechanisms but are weaker in the development of explanatory theory. We would argue that an explanatory theory, which indicates why and how these effects are produced, is an important addition to the usefulness of such findings.[1] These systematic reviews are stronger in their assessment of change outcomes, searching for evidence of better 'outcomes' from the intervention (a criticism of qualitative studies might be the loose focus on assessing outcomes), but weaker in the exploration of change process, and how this process in turn may affect outcomes.

The difference between the biomedical and social science traditions in this field has been perhaps accentuated by the dominance of symbolic interpretive approaches within UK health care management research already alluded to. The gap would have been less if there had been a strong tradition of UK quantitative organizational research, which was closer to the triallist paradigm. As Oakley (2001) points out, some social scientists in other settings do work in a more quasi-experimental way, drawing for instance on the pioneering work of Donald Campbell in the USA. Quasi-experimentalism is, however, very poorly represented in UK health management research.

There are some interesting qualitative studies on EBHC implementation already available, which conceive of the core problem in a very different light. Lomas' analysis (1993) of attempts to disseminate synthesized evidence into paediatric care in Canadian health care begins to unpick the 'black box' of how research enters into clinical

---

[1] The usefulness of theory development is an issue of contention between Oakley (2000), who sees theorizing as a potential vehicle for academic imperialism, and Pawson and Tilley (1997), who argue that the development of theory usefully provides more informed explanations of otherwise limited empirical observations.

practice. Here we have a single case study that generates a broader thematic discussion. Lomas recognizes that there are various routes by which research can reach clinical practice, including such varied mechanisms as informal education, regulatory review, and incentive structures. Lomas (1993: 444) argues that research information

must be carefully embedded in multiple routes of evidence in order to pressure practitioners into applying it to patient care.

It may be better to use multiple methods rather than search for a single change lever. Moreover, pressure to adopt evidence-based practice may be applied not solely by purposeful and designed 'interventions' but more diffusely by various pre-existing interest groups (such as community organizations with an interest in the health care issue in question). Lomas argues that a situational analysis should be undertaken to identify the most receptive organizations for evidence-based change, which he defines as those that

1. have an appreciation for 'classes of evidence' and the importance of research in determining clinical practice;
2. perceive that there is a problem in the reflection of research evidence in clinical practices for children;
3. perceive themselves as having a role in minimizing this problem;
4. have structures and mechanisms in place, which they are willing to use to influence practitioners.

Here is a holistic analysis, which considers the world of clinical practice as a whole and identifies a range of possible influence mechanisms on it, all of which may be important. It uses a different form of case-study-based evidence from quasi-experimental evidence. It suggests that the decision to adopt may 'tip' once sufficient multiple pressures are in place and where the context has sufficient levels of receptivity.

A set of articles has appeared in a recent issue of *Health Care Management Review*, which generally uses qualitative and case-study-based methods. The articles seek to explore how evidence is, or is not, incorporated within clinical practice. A common theme within this suite of papers is that the reception of evidence is strongly influenced by the nature of the underlying health care system, such as its ability to learn and create knowledge (Lemieux-Charles et al. 2002), the perceptions of the benefits and risks to different interest groups associated with an innovation (Denis et al. 2002), and the social distribution of legitimacy and credibility (Maguire 2002) of evidence and knowledge production, including shifts in such distributions. Curiously, this stream of literature has been mainly developed by Canadian researchers, although we also produced a UK-based paper in this edition (Dopson et al. 2002).

We conclude that an important 'gap' in the present EBHC implementation literature in the UK is a need for more sustained interpretive work, which explores the role and motives of actors and the influence of the organizational context and the social construction of evidence in much greater light. Existing work in this area is discussed in detail in Chapter 3.

2.7 High organizational complexity and variability: implications for EBHC implementation

Our overall perspective is that the process of EBHC implementation can be usefully seen as a decision stream being processed (along with many other competing issues) by the health care organizations charged with its implementation. In this respect, EBHC is no different from alternative issues that try to rise up against the agenda of health care organizations, such as quality management or the retention of financial control. EBHC implementation has to attract resources, time, and sustained attention if it is to succeed. While the corporate level of health care organizations can adopt evidence-based practice as a formal policy, it only becomes real if it is enacted by a large number of front-line clinical groups over which senior management has limited control. The issue has to be owned by the front-line clinical groups before substantial change in clinical practice can be secured.

The organizational domain in which EBHC sits is both complex, exhibiting interacting forces that, taken together, importantly affect decision outcomes, and variable as the balance of these forces differs markedly from one setting to another. This complexity and variability may be fateful in influencing the career of EBHC initiatives. In our view, the following dimensions of organizational complexity—and sources of variability—need to be addressed.

2.7.1 *The importance of context*

We argue that organizational change processes—of which a shift to evidence-based practice is but one example—are highly context-dependent and not at all generic in nature. Such processes are likely to vary strongly from one health care organization to another. Therefore an identification and analysis of 'context' has to be part of any full account. On the other hand, we do not wish to argue that every context is different and no patterning at all can be discerned, because of infinite micro variability. We seek to establish some core factors, which produce low-level patterning even if not predictive laws. So what might be the main dimensions of context? Firstly, context varies across time and space so that results from one country cannot be easily exported to another country where the health care system is different (studies in the USA may only have partial direct relevance to the National Health Service [NHS]), nor results from an earlier time period extrapolated to a later time period when there may be different roles, relationships, and power bases apparent within the health care system (so trade unions had far more power in the NHS of the 1970s than that of the 1990s).

Secondly, there may be intersectoral differences, which affect the process of EBHC implementation. Acute care/primary care (AC/PC) and mental health settings may all display distinctive patterns of roles, relationships, and working practices. Acute settings can be seen as the most directly managed and as having strong, distinct, clinical specialities. By contrast, community health services act more as loosely coupled 'networks' (Flynn et al. 1996), where managerial authority is weak and multidisciplinary 'communities of practice' (Wenger 1998) are more evident. Mental health settings may also display a pattern of stronger multidisciplinary working, which enables evidence to cross professional boundaries more easily. While we do not present any mental health examples in this book, we do draw both on acute sector and primary care examples so that intersectoral comparison will be interesting.

Thirdly, there may be subtly different histories, cultures, patterns of roles and relationships, and capability for learning and change (Pettigrew et al. 1992) apparent from one setting to another. Taken together, this suggests some contexts are much more 'receptive' to EBHC ideas than others in broader ways than simply attitudes to evidence (Lomas 1993); notably we would be interested to locate any 'high change–high learning' settings that are more readily able to absorb new information and use it to produce local change.

We conclude that EBHC-based change interventions are unlikely to have generic effects, but remain highly context-dependent. This is a different position from that evident in the mainstream EBHC implementation literature, which is more concerned to assess the generic impact of EBHC-related change interventions across a variety of contexts. Nevertheless, we need to specify the core dimensions of context that influence the career of EBHC innovations with some precision, in order to escape from the charge that 'everything is different'. Hence the rather descriptive discussion of elements of context that influence the career of EBHC ideas documented in Section 5.3 in this book.

2.7.2 *Processes, not events*

A second dimension of complexity lies in the assessment of the change outcome. EBHC implementation cannot be judged in a simple, binary manner according to whether it has been implemented or not. The outcome indicator, in other words, is complex. The extent to which an innovation has been adopted in practice requires a fine judgement based on a detailed knowledge of clinical practices (rather than a mere change in formal organizational policy). Such implementation should be seen as a continuing process rather than as a discrete event: for example, early adoption of an EBHC innovation such as a new drug may be followed by later 'unadoption', in whole or in part. One's conclusion about the degree of adoption is sensitive to the point in time at which it is made. So we need a longitudinal perspective that enables us to trace the career of the EBHC innovation over a long period. There are possible change outcomes, which should be explored (such as partial adoption, modified adoption, and pretence of adoption or local customization), as well as a simple adoption–non-adoption dichotomy.

2.7.3 *The contestability of evidence*

In some instances, the evidence base that supports an EBHC innovation may be extremely well founded, such as a meta-analysis across a number of RCTs which finds a consistent effect. Many EBHC innovations do not display this level of evidence and are hence highly contestable. Even if one stays within the triallist paradigm, the number of well-conducted trials into a particular treatment or intervention may be highly limited, as might the populations to whom the trial results are scientifically applicable, or the results may be inconclusive or even contradictory. Different professional groups tend to cite studies that suit them and ignore those that do not. There may be controversies between different scientific camps, which evolve over time, as new bits of evidence come to light. The contestable nature of evidence is even greater as one broadens out from the RCT paradigm and uses evidence drawn from different methods, some of which will be favoured by certain interest groups.

2.7.4 *Multiple actors*

A fourth important dimension of complexity is the large number of agencies and occupational groups often involved in EBHC implementation. The different agencies include primary health care organizations, acute health care organizations, central government, civil servants, and specialist research agencies. The occupational groups include doctors (consultants and GPs), nurses (hospital nurses and primary care nurses), allied health professionals (AHPs), HSRs, general managers, and user representatives in such fields as maternity services or mental health care (Ferlie et al. 2002). It is a 'crowded field', having a wide range of organizations and interest groups, often with different priorities and agendas. Many EBHC-based innovations seek to disturb a division of labour traditionally agreed across occupational groups, such as the division of labour between doctors and nurses (typically by delegating more routine tasks from medicine to nursing or from secondary care to primary care). The boundaries between these occupational groups may be very difficult to cross in practice. It is also the case that the degree of occupational complexity varies from one innovation to another with some EBHC innovations being more focal (with one dominant stakeholder) and others more diffuse (with a range of stakeholders). Many EBHC innovations, however, appear to involve a large range of stakeholders. We need to be aware of the different actors present in any implementation process and identify any intergroup boundaries that the innovation needs to cross to secure implementation.

2.7.5 *Autonomous professional groupings*

Autonomous professional groupings are not simply conventional occupational groups, but often well-established professions. This is a further source of complexity and variability. The professionalized organization has traditionally been seen as presenting singular dynamics (Freidson 1970; Mintzberg 1983) in which elite professional groupings (notably clinicians) dominate the organizations that nominally employ them. Other groups (such as nurses) are also engaged in a professionalization project, but have not as yet secured the power base of medicine. The retention of autonomy over working practices represents a core value for elite professionals, and suggests a limited role for conventional forms of managerial control and external instruction. Professionals also seek to establish 'jurisdictions' (Abbott 1988) and defend their turf from encroachment by other professional groups, which again acts as an innovation 'blocker'. Whether EBHC is seen as being driven by a particular professional group will impact on how it is received by that group.

2.7.6 *Cognitive boundaries: different research paradigms*

Professional groupings may display different research cultures, agendas, and questions. They have a cognitive as well as a social element. The cognitive element to 'acceptable' and legitimated forms of knowledge is important within science-based organizations, including health care (Beck 1992; Whitley 2000).

Are all health care professionals guided by the classic Mertonian norms (Merton 1973), which attribute a communalistic, universalistic, and disinterested character to scientific knowledge? Within this account, biomedical knowledge should have a generally accepted character and should hence spread widely across a field sharing a common epistemology. Against this, the research 'paradigm' concept (Kuhn 1970; Oakley 2001) suggests that a discipline with developed paradigmatic status displays distinct cognitive assumptions. Paradigms may not only be different but incommensurable, advancing different claims to knowledge (Burrell and Morgan 1979). Their adherents 'talk past' each other, lacking common ground for productive dialogue and at worst producing paradigm wars (Oakley 2001). Beck (1992) argues that a process of increased scientific differentiation leads to surplus knowledge production and 'hypercomplexity', which paradoxically enables the end-user of research to exercise more choice between a growing number of plausible knowledge claims. One possibility is that an increased number of professionalized or professionalizing occupations go on to produce distinctive research styles and particular bodies of knowledge that are not seen as authoritative within other paradigms and professionally influenced research cultures.

2.8   Methodological implications: a finely grained approach to analysing EBHC initiatives

We argue that EBHC is likely to be imperfectly implemented within such highly complex and variable settings characteristic of health care. Moreover, it is not simple to define the change outcome in terms of the adoption of changed clinical behaviours, which are better aligned with evidence. Such an assessment may indeed vary according to the point in time at which it is made. So adoption may be followed by unadoption or customization. Different stakeholders may have different views about the extent to which change has been achieved within practice, as opposed to being declared formal policy. The nature and quality of the decision-making process may influence the change outcome, however it is defined, and analysis should try to unpack any process–outcome linkages.

Some important methodological implications arise from these observations. This perspective suggests the need for finely grained and holistic analyses of the process of EBHC implementation within real-life clinical settings. The *how* and *why* questions of EBHC moving into practice are important as well as the *what* questions. The 'how' question indeed shapes the 'what' outcome. There is a need for a longitudinal element to investigation so that the career of the EBHC innovation can be plotted over time, and snapshot analyses may be highly misleading. It certainly calls for a form of pluralistic evaluation combining formal and informal evaluation, whereby the perspectives of a range of stakeholders are accessed and presented.

2.9   Concluding remarks

This chapter has argued that the process of EBHC implementation needs to be understood within its broader organizational studies context. This begs the question of what sort of organizational analytic framework should be employed. Three of the main traditions in organizational analysis were briefly outlined, which distinguished between modernist, symbolic interpretive, and postmodernist perspectives. We placed ourselves broadly in the symbolic interpretive tradition. We noted that the symbolic interpretive tradition appears to be strongly represented in mainstream UK health management literature, although it displays some weaknesses, such as a lack of a strong connection to theory and weak external validity. The more specific literature on EBHC implementation has mainly used techniques drawn from the biomedical, triallist, paradigm, and symbolic interpretive approaches that have been less well developed (although some work in this tradition has been evident). Our intention in this monograph is to add further to this symbolic interpretive literature on EBHC implementation, and to do this with an explicit concern for theory and for higher levels of external validity.

The triallist literature on EBHC implementation has somewhat neglected the organizational domain as an unexplored residual or an 'effect modifier'. Its concern has been above all to identify change interventions that 'work', irrespective of their organizational context. We argue by contrast, that the organizational domain is both complex and variable and that it affects EBHC implementation in important ways. So an appreciation of context is as important as a knowledge of 'mechanism' in the explanation of outcomes, as Pawson and Tilly (1997) argue in their model of realistic evaluation. This is an unsurprising conclusion in terms of organizational research but relatively novel in the world of EBHC, which has only more recently engaged with organizational forms of analysis.

In Chapters 7 and 8 we describe how EBHC moves into practice. We will emphasize that EBHC is 'enacted' in particular work settings by the actions of decision-makers in day-to-day life (Weick 1995). This is in turn linked to an active process of 'sense-making' by socially reflexive agents who generate mechanisms and routines that enable them to construct an appreciation of environmental forces (Porac et al. 1989; Weick 1995). The cognitive basis of behavioural change is important here. In the EBHC case, agents may be seen to interpret imperfect, contested, and competing forms of formal evidence and weigh up their relevance for the particular work setting in which they are embedded. There are powerful 'communities of practice' (Wenger 1998) (such as clinical teams or indeed specialities) that operate at a small group level, processing evidence and turning it into decisions about changes to work routines. These communities of practice may have idiosyncratic views about what constitutes compelling evidence. There may also be barriers to the effective translation of evidence across the boundaries that exist between different communities of practices. Our next chapter, however, describes in more detail the concept of EBHC and what is known about the so-called 'implementation gap'.

3

Evidence-Based Health Care and the Implementation Gap

Sue Dopson, Louise Locock, John Gabbay, Ewan Ferlie, and Louise Fitzgerald

3.1 Introduction

Evidence-based policy (EBP) and practice are now in vogue across a wide range of government departments and academic disciplines, including education, social care, management, and criminology (Davies et al. 1999; Trinder and Reynolds 2000; Black 2001). Government initiatives that aim to take forward the 'modernizing' government agenda have confirmed the central role that evidence is expected to play in policy-making for the twenty-first century. Given this flurry of interest and coverage, it is easy to overlook the fact that welfare policy has a long and distinguished history of being informed by research evidence. (See the work of Brian Abel-Smith, Charles Booth, and Seebohm Rowntree.)

Despite some diverse exemplification, there is widespread common agreement on some basic underpinnings of evidence-based practice agenda (perhaps better termed evidence-informed or even evidence-aware):

1. There should be some agreement as to what counts as evidence in what circumstances.
2. There should be a strategy of creating evidence in priority areas, with concomitant systematic efforts to accumulate evidence in the form of robust bodies of knowledge.
3. Such evidence should be actively disseminated to where it is most needed, and made available for the widest possible use.
4. Strategies should be put in place to ensure the integration of evidence into policy and encourage the utilization of evidence in practice.

Notwithstanding the considerable efforts expended across the public sector on the EBP agenda, the approach has received some sustained critique as well as provoking some disillusionment about a lack of deep-rooted impact (Davies and Boruch 2001; Trinder and Reynolds 2000). In particular, some progress on items 1–3 above has thrown into sharp relief the difficulties of achieving item 4: improved research utilization.

Policy players and service delivery managers are recognizing that devising better mechanisms for pushing research information out (dissemination) is having only limited success and are seeking more effective ways of implementing evidence-based practice. In addition, research commissioners are paying increasing attention to how the work they commission is utilized, and are insisting that researchers pay far greater attention to their potential user audience. Evidence-based medicine (EBM) was one of the first manifestations of the preoccupation with EBP and has exercised enormous influence both within health care and across policy more generally. This chapter seeks to explore the reasons for the emergence and impact of EBM, more recently referred to as evidence-based health care (EBHC), and to understand some of the factors that have affected its uptake. It acts as an important background chapter for the subsequent presentation of empirical evidence.

As already mentioned in the introduction in Chapter 2, many early enthusiasts of EBHC naïvely assumed that the case for implementation would be self-evident and that it would spread automatically and quickly. This assumption was based on the notion that research evidence was incontestable and that robust evidence would be used by practitioners because it would self-evidently improve clinical practice and clinical outcomes. Such thoughts have had to be revised as the complexities of implementation have been acknowledged, notably the continued autonomy and dominance of the medical profession and the strong influence of the biomedical science model on what is considered legitimate evidence. We begin by examining the nature of EBHC.

3.2 What is EBHC?

It is argued that EBHC represents a paradigm shift, from medical practice based on the accumulation of clinical observation, expertise, and experience towards one characterized by a systematic search for rigorous and relevant scientific evidence (EBM Working Group 1992).

Table 3.1 contrasts the components of the so-called 'new' paradigm with the 'old' paradigm.

Davidoff and colleagues are amongst many writers who seek to identify the components of an evidence-based approach. They identify five linked ideas as central to EBHC:

Firstly, clinical decisions should be based on the best available scientific evidence; secondly, the clinical problem—rather than habits or protocols—should determine the type of evidence to be sought; thirdly, identifying the best evidence means using epidemiological and biostatistical ways of thinking; fourthly, conclusions derived from identifying and critically appraising evidence are useful only if put into action in managing patients or making health care decisions; and, finally, performance should be constantly evaluated. (Davidoff et al. 1995: 1085)

A key underlying assumption of EBHC is that not all evidence is equivalent. There is a hierarchy of study design in terms of the strength they provide. In the forefront of the list is the randomized control trial (RCT); non-randomized controlled studies and case stud-

Table 3.1   *The former and new paradigm of evidence-based medicine (EBM)*

• Unsystematic observations from clinical experience are a valid way of building and maintaining one's knowledge about patient prognosis, the value of diagnostic tests, and the efficacy of treatments	• Whilst clinical experience and the development of clinical instincts are a crucial part of becoming a competent physician, information derived from clinical experience and intuition must be interpreted cautiously, for it may be misleading
• The study and understanding of basic mechanisms of disease and patho-physiological principles are a sufficient guide for clinical practice	• The study and understanding of basic mechanisms of disease are necessary but insufficient guides for clinical practice. The rationales for diagnosis and treatment, which follow from basic pathophysiological principles, may in fact be incorrect, leading to inaccurate predictions about the performance of diagnostic tests and the efficacy of treatment
• A combination of thorough traditional medical training and common sense is sufficient to allow one to evaluate new tests and treatments	
• Content expertise and clinical experience are a sufficient base from which to generate valid guidelines for clinical practice	• Understanding certain rules of evidence, especially sound epidemiological and/or experimental design, is necessary to correctly interpret literature on causation, prognosis, diagnostic tests, and treatment strategy

ies occupy a lower position in the hierarchy. The systematic reviews carried out by the Cochrane Collaboration seek to draw together evidence from all rigorously conducted trials on a particular topic, so that practice is not based simply on the results of one trial (Davis et al. 1992, 1995; Grimshaw and Russel 1993; Sheldon and Chalmers 1994; Chalmers and Altman 1995; Deeks et al. 1996 Guide to Systematic Reviews 1996).

EBM and EBHC have sometimes been criticized for reducing clinical practice to 'cookbook medicine', following a recipe rather than exercising clinical judgement. However, Sackett and colleagues seek to demonstrate how external research evidence should support clinical judgement, rather than replace it. EBM, they argue, is

the conscientious, explicit and judicious use of current best evidence in making decisions about the care of individual patients. . . . It requires a bottom-up approach that integrates the best external evidence with individual clinical expertise and patients' choice. . . . External clinical evidence can inform, but can never replace, individual clinical expertise, and it is this expertise that decides whether external evidence applies to the individual patient at all and, if so, how it should be integrated into a clinical decision. (Sackett et al. 1996: 71)

EBM, they continue,

is not restricted to randomised trials and meta-analyses. It involves tracking down the best external evidence with which to answer our clinical questions. . . . It is when asking questions about therapy that we should try to avoid the non-experimental approaches, since these routinely lead to false-positive conclusions about efficacy. Because the randomised trial, and especially the systematic review of several randomised trials, is so much more likely to inform us and so much less likely to mislead us, it has become the 'gold standard' for judging whether a treatment does more good than harm. . . . If no randomised trial has been carried out for our patient's predicament, we must follow the trail to the next best external evidence and work from there.

3.3 The rationale for EBHC: the gap between research and practice

Problems in translating evidence into clinical practice are not new. An early example of delayed uptake of innovations is the use of lemon juice to prevent scurvy. James Lancaster demonstrated its effectiveness in 1601, but it was not until 1747 that James Lind repeated the experiment, and the British Navy did not fully adopt the innovation until 1795, and in the case of the merchant marines, 1865 (Mosteller 1981).

In recent decades medical research has dramatically increased the amount of evidence and range of treatment options available. Despite this rapid growth in what medical technology and research can offer, the medical literature is littered with examples of research findings that have not found timely acceptance in practice. Indeed, the proliferation of new medical knowledge and techniques is precisely one reason why clinical practice is characterized by substantial variations, as practitioners struggle to keep abreast of advances.

The problem has been succinctly described by Lomas and Haynes (1988: 77):

In an ideal world, there would be no gap between what is known from sound research and the means to promote health and the means actually employed by health care practitioners in administering care to their patients. In fact, however, there is a distressing distance between health care knowledge in general and the practices of individual clinicians for most validated health care procedures.

3.4   The emergence of the EBHC movement

The EBHC movement emerged as a response to unacceptable variations in practice and failure to act on available evidence. The landmark book in 1971 by British epidemiologist Archibald Cochrane entitled *Effectiveness and Efficiency: Random Reflections on Health Services* proved to be an important catalyst (Cochrane 1971). Cochrane set out a case for the greater use of scientific techniques in health services research (HSR) as a way of achieving greater effectiveness and efficiency in patient care. He put forward two major steps. Firstly, policy-makers need to 'measure the effect of a particular medical action in altering the natural history of a particular disease for the better', usually in the context of an RCT, set up to determine the difference between a group with a given disease who are randomly assigned to a particular intervention and groups who are either given a standard treatment or no treatment at all. Cochrane defined this step as effectiveness. Secondly, personnel and resources needed to be applied optimally to achieve clinical effectiveness, resulting in efficiency. Throughout his book, Cochrane illustrates how care could be improved in a number of clinical areas, by using positive results from clinical trials to define practice.

Cochrane advocated setting up a new organization to independently assess and compare medical research. This took another two decades to achieve. In the meantime, individual research groups pioneered the approach he had outlined, notably a team in Oxford reviewing the evidence for effective care in pregnancy and childbirth (Chalmers et al. 1989). In the foreword to this book, Cochrane himself described the study as 'a real milestone in the history of randomized trials and in the evaluation of care', and suggested that other specialities should copy the methods used. Cochrane's proposed independent research evaluation body was eventually set up in 1993 in Oxford with the launch of the international Cochrane Collaboration, which has executed systematic reviews of the medical evidence. Since the launch, hundreds of systematic reviews have been completed. In ten years the Cochrane Collaboration has become a comprehensive global network of researchers and practitioners monitoring just over fifty areas of intervention of disease and medicine and related fields. The network is supported by fifteen communications centres of different sizes with methodological competence and infrastructure for automatic information handling.

The positive experience of the Cochrane Collaboration was one important impetus for the creation of the Campbell Collaboration, an international network of researchers, practitioners, and financiers for development, maintenance, and dissemination of systematic reviews of knowledge regarding the effects of contributions and social intervention programmes for social work, criminal justice, and education. The overall purpose of Campbell Collaboration is to make the combined experience of international research on effective measures, interventions, and programmes more readily available to practitioners and policy-makers and to take the responsibility for quality scrutiny of research contributions. This means that internationally expanding primary research is subjected to quality control scrutiny, research results are summarized and distributed to users, and assessment of the need of further primary research is considered.

Oxford is also home to the Centre for Evidence-Based Medicine at the John Radcliffe Hospital, led for many years by David Sackett, an American physician. Sackett and the Centre have played a major role in spreading understanding of EBHC and providing practical help in applying it, and in creating a focus for an enthusiastic group of doctors from the UK and other countries, especially North America, to exchange ideas.

3.4.1 *Interest from policy-makers*

The emergence of EBHC was largely professionally driven, although it took some time to become generally accepted and has not been uncontested within the medical profession—a point to which we return later. Over time, politicians, managers, and commissioners in both the USA and the UK began to take an interest in EBHC and to see it as the key to changing clinical practice and improving health care quality. They therefore began to seek ways to increase its uptake. In the UK these efforts have included projects to draft treatment guidelines for specific conditions, and a number of demonstration projects designed to change clinical practice in line with evidence. These were to generate lessons to be disseminated to the wider NHS (Dopson et al. 1999; Locock et al. 1999). New systems and organizations have been set up, devoted to the evaluation and dissemination of clinical evidence, such as the NHS Health Technology Assessment Programme (www.hta.nhsweb.nhs.uk), the Deeks et al. 1996 (www.york.ac.uk/inst/crd/welcome.htm), and the National Institute for Clinical Excellence (www.nice.org.uk/default-xmas.htm). Contact, Help, Advice, and Information Network for Effective Health Care (CHAIN) (www.nhsu.nhs.uk/chain/) is an informal email network for people working in health care with an interest in EBHC.

EBHC is also at the forefront of policy decisions in the health care systems of Europe and North America (Woolf et al. 1999). Searches on MEDLINE carried out in 2000 (Chambers 2000) found just one US article about EBM in 1995 and 1996, compared with a total of 294 over the next two years and roughly the same number for 1999 and 2000. In 1997, the Agency for Health Care Policy Research (now the Agency for Health Care Research and Quality) established twelve evidence-based practice centres around the USA intended to provide evidence reports on a variety of clinical treatments for dissemination and policy-making.

There are a number of possible explanations for policy-makers' interest in EBHC; one explanation is a genuine wish to improve the quality and consistency of care for patients. Alternatively, or in addition, different stakeholders will have their own agenda, priorities, and views about the potential value of EBHC.

Politicians, managers, and economists may see EBHC as a method of cutting costs while preserving standards of care, or as a way of justifying rationing decisions. Weisbrod (1991) has argued that health care consumer demand has only relatively recently increased to the point where strict attention to resource allocation is needed, and that advances in medical technology have increased pressure on resources. EBHC offers a means of ensuring maximally effective care, and of discarding ineffective practices and techniques, thereby making cost savings. Newer techniques may be less invasive and produce better outcomes, requiring shorter hospital stays and fewer follow-ups. However, EBHC as a way of cutting costs is firmly rejected by its advocates amongst the medical profession, who argue that raising the standard of practice may lead to increased expenditure (Sackett et al. 1996).

Managers may also perceive EBHC as a vehicle for increased control of doctors. Clinical autonomy and medical professional dominance have proved highly resistant to managerial and political intervention (Freidson 1989; Wolinsky 1993; Harrison 1999). EBHC may be seen as a way of moving away from medicine as a mysterious art form to one that can be codified, standardized, and made transparent. Klein (1996: 85) suggests:

[T]he new scientism appears to offer politicians less pain, less responsibility for taking difficult decisions and a legitimate way of curbing what are often seen as the idiosyncratic and extravagant practices of doctors.

Politicians may view EBHC as a lever through which to improve the population's perception of health services, to rally support for their political party and appeal to voters. There has been growing awareness of the need to improve accountability and demonstrate that public money is being spent wisely to the benefit of patients. The tie-in of EBM with 'New Labour' visions of an improved NHS is a good example of the political use of EBHC. The government White Paper *The New NHS* (Secretary of State 1997) signalled the use of EBHC as a way to improve standards of care for all citizens, and to respond to a number of high-profile malpractice scandals.

Whilst the engagement of policy-makers may increase the profile of EBHC and perhaps its influence and uptake, the shift away from a purely professionally driven movement towards a policy initiative may be something of a double-edged sword. The medical profession may react against the hijacking of EBHC by managerial and political concerns that they mistrust—a question to which we return below.

3.5   Can EBHC bridge the implementation gap?

The idea of an implementation deficit or gap between what is planned and what is actually achieved (raised in Chapter 2) has a long-standing place in the analysis of public policy (Pressman and Wildavsky 1973; Alford 1975) and in organizational studies of the diffusion of innovations (Rogers 1995; Van de Ven et al. 1999). In both fields it has long been argued that it is wrong to assume that change will be smooth, straightforward, and linear. Rather we can expect a negotiated process, in which resistance and challenge play an inevitable part. As Hogwood and Gunn (1984: 208) suggest:

Implementation must involve a process of interaction between organizations, the members of which may have different values, perspectives, and priorities from one another, and from those advocating the policy.

This will be especially true in a professionalized organization such as the NHS, in which interactions between different professional subgroups within each organization are just as important as relations between organizations.

EBHC represents something of a paradox. As stated earlier, ironically it has been assumed that evidence-based ways of thinking and behaving would diffuse in a linear and rational way. This assumption continued even in the face of clear empirical evidence that diffusion of specific pieces of research evidence was not happening in that way (Dopson and Gabbay 1995). Yet, paradoxically, despite this being precisely the problem that led to the need for EBHC, policy-makers and EBHC enthusiasts alike have frequently taken a somewhat simplistic view of the implementation gap they aim to address. Its advocates have sometimes been surprised at the degree of resistance to something that seems to them both self-evidently good and worthwhile, and also entirely consistent with the 'scientific' biomedical paradigm within which they operate.

For some time it was assumed that the implementation gap between research evidence and practice was a technical one of information availability—if information could be disseminated more efficiently, in a digestible form, changes in practice would automatically follow. Commentaries on EBM and EBHC routinely draw attention to factors such as information overload, the gap in skills needed to interpret research, and the need to invest in better, usually electronic, sources of evidence (Haines and Donald 1998; Gray 2001). It has become clear that reliance on passive diffusion of information to keep health professionals up to date is doomed to failure in a global environment in which around two million articles on medical issues are published annually (Mulrow 1994). Early pioneers of EBHC therefore targeted their efforts at ensuring that information was more readily accessible, for example in the form of guidelines and summaries of recent publications. Reviews of primary research have been provided by the Cochrane library, the Deeks et al. 1996, and the Health Technology Assessment Programme, amongst others. (These and other data sources are usefully reviewed in Gray 2001, Appendix 1, and are the heart of the nascent National Electronic Library for Health, which is designed to make it easier to access such evidence.)

EBHC is not, however, simply about getting specific pieces of research evidence into practice. It is about creating a culture where practitioners automatically think in an 'evidence'-based way every time they see a new case, where it becomes instinctive to seek out research evidence and base treatment decisions on that evidence. This requires an appreciation of the social context of which practioners are a part. Drawing on Aristotelian analysis of rhetoric, Van de Ven and Shomaker (2002) argue that EBHC has thus far concentrated on only one aspect of rhetorical persuasion, namely logos—the clarity and logic of the argument and its supporting evidence. Effective rhetoric, however, also relies on pathos—the power to stir the emotions, beliefs, values, knowledge, and imagination of the audience and generate empathy, and ethos—the credibility, legitimacy, and authority of the speaker (Barnes 1995). Van de Ven and Shomaker (2002: 91) conclude:

To be successful at this mission, proponents of EBHC must, as Aristotle exhorts, have the ability to reason logically, understand human character and goodness in their various forms so as to be a creditable witness, and understand human emotions so as to better appreciate the beliefs and experiences of others.

The individual and collective reactions of doctors themselves to the rhetoric of EBHC are thus crucial in understanding its impact. These reactions have been mixed, and have changed over time; analysis of medicine's response helps explain both why EBHC has had as much impact as it has, and why it has sometimes been resisted and rejected. This brings us to the heart of medicine's image of itself and of its scientific basis, relations within the profession, the perennial question of power and autonomy, and the profession's relations with managers, policy-makers, and other professionals.

Greenhalgh et al. (2004: 25), in a systematic review of the literature on diffusion, dissemination, and sustainability of innovations in health service delivery and organization, argue that because of the highly contextual and contingent nature of the process of spread and sustainability, it was not possible for them to make formulaic, universally applicable recommendations for practice and policy.

Although the emphasis in the text that follows is on the problems and barriers which EBHC has faced, it would be entirely wrong to imply it had had no effect. Of all the different versions of EBP and evidence-based practice in different disciplines, EBHC has undoubtedly been one of the most successful (Davies et al. 1999). However, because the change in attitudes towards it and its impact on policy have been gradual, it is easy to forget just how radical it seemed in its early days. Over the ten years since our research in this field began, EBHC has evolved from a contested minority pursuit to a new orthodoxy—at least outwardly. Nonetheless, although the principle of EBHC has largely been accepted, practice still does not necessarily reflect this—it is the reasons for this continuing discrepancy between, for example, what doctors say, what they think, and what they actually do that we seek to understand.

The degree of influence that EBHC has enjoyed so far can be attributed largely to two factors. One is the fact that it was largely professionally driven in its early stages—although it has since been taken up by policy-makers and managers—and the other factor is EBHC's appeal to a biomedical scientific agenda.

Given all the evidence that doctors respond most readily to peer influence, peer comparison, and peer example (Hiss et al. 1978; West et al. 1999; Locock et al. 2001), professional leadership has, in the end, been one of EBHC major strengths. In general, our suite of studies found widespread support for the application of EBHC as redefined by Sackett, as illustrated by this quotation from an associate adviser in general practice:

David Sackett defused a lot of criticism very well by defining EBHC as a bottom-up approach based on good clinical management and supported by the best available evidence and taking into account patient priorities. (Fitzgerald et al. 1999)

Support, in principle, for EBHC did not necessarily mean, however, that it was being applied in day-to-day practice as one general practitioner (GP) described:

There should be EBM. Most of the things I do, I try to think of a reason why I am doing it, though I am not able to recall the evidence or where it has come from. I have a faint memory or I have read something and I obviously can't remember where I have read them. (Dawson et al. 1998)

From the same study, a registrar commented:

We are just too busy to be able to stop on a ward round and discuss evidence-based medicine for every patient—it's inappropriate. Nice in principle but difficult to do in practice.

Despite current acceptance of the idea, early resistance was often more overtly hostile. Our research in the late 1990s revealed apocryphal stories of deep resentment towards the leaders of the EBHC movement. As one sardonic medical clinical director put it: 'We're creating an industry to worship the great god [of EBM]' (CSAG 1998). Pioneers of EBHC were sometimes heavily criticized by other doctors threatened by the challenge to their established practice, and for a while were operating too far beyond the norms of some of their colleagues to gain widespread credibility and acceptance. Most doctors are unlikely to be persuaded while the message is seen to come from a few mavericks.

I go to the occasional academic meeting but the trouble with those is that you get speakers who tend to have a hobby horse and although briefly you can believe what they are saying, on the whole it fades away within a few days unless it is backed up by genuine numbers of other people saying the same thing. (Consultant interviewee, Wood et al. 1998)

One common group of negative reactions argued that medical care had always been evidence-based, and that EBHC was therefore neither new nor necessary. Indeed, it was perceived as insulting to be told that one's practice was not evidence-based—this despite all the research demonstrating variations in practice and failure to act on new evidence. This reaction can be partly understood by exploring different understandings of the word 'evidence', as illustrated by the following quotations from a medical director and consultant respectively:

Published articles are usually contentious. You need a forum to discuss them, to gather information, to dissect them, to say 'it works OK in a teaching hospital, but would it work here in a DGH [district general hospital]?', to ask whether they'll stand the test of time.... What gets me is our practice has always been based on evidence—I don't just get out of bed in the morning and look out of the window and think 'what shall I do today?'—but it's *practical* evidence, based on knowing what's happening, not on working it out statistically. (Locock et al. 1999)

We all practice EBHC because we collect our evidence from different sources and apply our own filter to produce the best answer. We may get it slightly wrong, but I don't honestly believe we get it any more wrong than relying on published data. (Dawson et al. 1998)

This is further borne out by the work of Fairhurst and Huby (1998) examining how GPs negotiate the implementation of evidence. The authors identify a distinction between 'trial data'—the pure scientific research findings—and 'practical knowledge'. GPs make judgements about the meaning and applicability of trial data in the context of other sources of evidence, including their own experience, the advice of respected hospital colleagues, and local norms of practice. From this emerges a form of practical, applied knowledge.

The focus on alternative forms of evidence has led to a more subtle critique of EBHC. Whilst accepting that medicine has not always been based on research evidence and that EBHC is indeed a new and necessary way of looking at things, this critique suggests that it has an overly rigid and reductionist emphasis on scientific evidence as the primary determinant of clinical practice.

This reaction throws light on the perennial tension between medicine as art or craft, and medicine as science (Hunter 1996). EBHC is entirely consonant with, and a product of, the biomedical model, and therefore holds a powerful attraction to doctors trained in that model. As Klein (1996: 85) says, 'who, after all, can be against science? . . . Who can do anything but welcome the prospect of weeding out interventions that appear to be based on faith and tradition rather than evidence?' Williamson (1992) and Hunter (1996) argue that the arrival of EBM and EBHC may serve to reinforce the long-standing hierarchical distinction between the quantifiable and measurable facts of research evidence and the 'mere knowledge' of clinical practice, which draws on an anecdotal and unscientific evidence base.

Yet doctors are also conscious of the complexity and uncertainty of much medical decision-making, the heterogeneity of patients, the importance of other factors such as socio-economic circumstances and co-morbidity, and the difficulty of extrapolating research results to the wider population and to different local contexts. One consultant argued:

I think it is a complete hoax personally . . . trials are done on such specific, clean questions but they never quite apply to the patient in front of you. . . . I think that is the problem with practice at my level—it is very individual. That is why I don't agree with EBM: there isn't any evidence to help you deal with the difficult patient. (Dawson et al. 1998)

The 'imposition of a spurious rationality on a sometimes inherently irrational process' (McKee and Clarke 1995) is seen to undervalue medicine's more holistic and empathic side, in which judgement, experience, and skill play an important part. The appeal to logic and science may fail if the rhetoric does not also engage with deeply held values and beliefs. As a clinical nurse specialist put it, 'You don't win on the basis of evidence, but on the basis of emotion. Until we address the emotional component of scientific—or pseudo-scientific—judgements, we won't achieve change' (Locock et al. 1999).

Goodman (2000) argues that 'EBM is in danger of becoming a new and unchallengeable orthodoxy following its own political agenda'; although its aim was to challenge the 'opinionated dogma of the expert' with something more rational, it risks creating a new source of dogma, which may be resented by its target audience, and fails to acknowledge the realities of daily clinical practice. As Armstrong (2002) suggests:

A tension...emerges between the maintenance of the autonomy of the profession as a collectivity through the promotion of a therapeutic rationality and the maintenance of the autonomy of the individual practitioner through the rhetoric of patient-centredness.

Inevitably, however, the idea of a dichotomy between art and science is too simplistic. Klein (1996: 85) suggests that 'like all evangelists, the enthusiasts for the new scientism are occasionally carried away by their sense of mission. But like all good scientists, they are also careful to stress that scientific knowledge can only be one input in decision-making'. Sackett's own definition cited towards the beginning of this chapter clearly allows for different kinds of information to influence clinical decisions, not just research evidence. The problem is one of perception and emphasis more than real content. In trying to shift the balance more in favour of the scientific side, EBHC has sometimes been perceived as going too far and stressing science to the exclusion of all else. EBHC is, for example, only likely to be accepted by doctors if they feel confident that it embraces both the scientific and more craft-based aspects of medical identity.

Despite successive attempts by managers, civil servants, and politicians to constrain medical power, doctors retain a striking degree of individual clinical autonomy, control over resources, and power over professional entry and regulation (Harrison 1999). Medical power, as we will see in Chapter 6, can help explain the implementation gap in three respects. Firstly, as has been documented in many studies of change in the setting of the NHS, doctors simply have power to resist any change they see as a threat, or as an extra burden of work. The fact that EBHC has been professionally led has helped limit this resistance, and as it has become more widely accepted, doctors have tailored their practice to conform, as these interviewees noted (Locock et al. 1999):

What makes me change—it's not scientific, but when I know what my peers are doing. We meet, we talk, we look at publications. (Medical director)

If the information is easily available, some people will change. When sufficient numbers of informed people make changes in their practice then peer pressure will make the rest change. (GP)

Secondly, however, such collective change can allow doctors to subvert EBHC. We have found, for example, doctors using the momentum of the EBHC movement to bring about changes in practice, which may improve the quality of patient experience, even though the evidence for the change is in fact not particularly strong (see Chapter 5 where we focus on context as an active part of the implementation process). Equally there are examples of using the rhetoric of EBHC to reject unwanted change. One nurse, for example, noted how doctors now use arguments such as:

'oh it's only one trial' and 'our patients aren't similar to those in the trial', which are the kinds of things they're learning to say, paradoxically, now that they're getting more into evidence-based medicine. (Dopson et al. 1999)

Thirdly, and more specifically, EBHC has been seen as one of many threats to traditional clinical autonomy, and this has undoubtedly provoked some resistance. Many clinicians in our studies have argued that EBHC strips them of the right to make medical decisions without challenge, and that it reduces clinical practice to following a set of codified instructions of protocols, which may be inappropriate for individual patients.

Show me a man with a rigid policy and I'll show you an idiot. (Consultant interviewee, Wood et al. 1998)

Evidence-based guidelines contribute in several ways to deprofessionalization (Haug 1973), including enabling patients to challenge and monitor doctors' decision-making more authoritatively; demystifying medicine as an art; relegating the doctor from professional to technical status; making doctors more easily subject to managerial control; and increasing litigation.

This is not to say, however, that doctors resist all guidelines. An important distinction may be whether doctors see them as authoritative, credible, professional documents that help them improve their practice, or as a form of management imposition and control. This often depends on the provenance of the guidelines.

The continuing complexity of health care and the need for clinical expertise in both drawing up and applying guidelines might suggest that fears of deprofessionalization are misplaced. A more plausible explanation would seem to be Freidson's stratification theory (1989). This suggests that collectively the medical profession retains power and freedom to determine its own practice, and is successfully fending off managerial control. However, this is achieved by developing a supervisory hierarchy within the profession itself, so that individual doctors' practice is reviewed and managed by other doctors. EBHC and the use of guidelines to regulate practice could be seen as a classic example of stratification, in which some doctors with 'expert' status sift the evidence and provide guidance for other doctors to put into practice. This may still be irksome and resisted to some extent, but may be more acceptable than managerial control, provided that the credibility and motivation of the experts is not in doubt (CSAG 1998).

The rhetoric of EBHC may be less acceptable, however, if it is perceived as tainted by a management agenda, which is largely about controlling costs. As noted earlier, managers and policy-makers have increasingly taken an interest in EBHC and may see it as a way of making savings, justifying rationing, and curbing clinical freedom.

The trouble is the move to use the phrase 'evidence-based medicine' has really come from a desire, a need, to be using money as effectively as possible and that still tends to get in the way quite a lot because it just does not fit with good medical practice. (GP/GP tutor, Fitzgerald et al. 1999)

I think it has been pounced on by the politicians and administrators as a way of saving money because they assume everything we do is totally useless. (Consultant, Dawson et al. 1998)

Klein (1996) argues that medical enthusiasts for EBHC are not the main problem, because they at least understand the complexity of medical decision-making and the need to consider research evidence alongside other clinical factors. The real danger, he concludes, is

that the rhetoric of a science-based NHS is likely to arouse excessive and unrealizable expectations . . . that a vulgarized form of the new scientism will be taken up by ministers and managers—and that their eventual disillusionment will lead to a disproportionate reaction. (Klein 1996: 85)

The problems here are twofold: firstly, doctors may turn against EBHC if they see it as a managerialist cost-cutting initiative; and secondly, policy-makers themselves may also reject EBHC when it fails to provide the easy, certain answers they seek to the intractable problems of complex health care decision-making.

Much of our research into the implementation of EBHC has explored the impact of local contextual factors in promoting or inhibiting its uptake. To some extent this is a different level of explanation of reactions to EBHC, which has less to do with generic features of medicine as a profession and its relationship with other parts of the system, and more to do with the minutiae of individual relationships, the past history, culture, and working patterns of each local organization, availability of resources, individual incentives and disincentives to change, project management arrangements, and the presence or absence of local opinion leaders who support the change (Dopson et al. 2002). This is a familiar litany from the generic change management and organizational behaviour literature. Any change initiative within health care organizations, not just EBHC, will be affected by a similar range of factors.

As argued in Chapter 2, the importance of local contextual factors, however, has consistently been overlooked by proponents of EBHC. Lemieux-Charles et al. (2002) argue that the literature on evidence-based decision-making has failed to draw on the large body of knowledge generated from social sciences, while the social science literature has not been systematically examined and synthesized for its applicability to health care. Over time, as it has become apparent that implementation would not be rational and linear, the EBHC movement has started to focus on the organizational and behavioural barriers to getting research into practice (Bero et al. 1998; Haines and Donald 1998). Researchers have struggled to find predictable levers, which can be relied upon to change practice successfully in any setting, using experimental methods to test their effectiveness. The Cochrane Collaboration Effective Practice and Organisation of Care Group (EPOC), for example, routinely restricts its selection criteria for systematic reviews of organizational interventions to RCTs, controlled clinical trials, controlled before and after studies, and interrupted time series analyses. Our findings, as discussed in subsequent chapters of this book, suggest that such an approach, based on the biomedical paradigm, is unlikely to provide reliable and helpful insights into organizational change.

Explanations for the biomedical mindset of so much recent research into the implementation of EBHC can be sought within the biomedical model, which has informed EBHC thinking. The day-to-day rhetoric of EBHC accepts a high degree of predictability and generalizability of well-founded research evidence. It relies on the assumption that systematic review of RCTs will provide reasonable certainty about what works and what does not, and that this will be generally true across all relevant patients.

Setting aside any long-standing epistemological arguments about the nature of scientific knowledge (Lakatos and Musgrave 1970), there is difficulty in sustaining this view of scientific clinical practice. As outlined above, one of the criticisms of EBHC is that diagnosis and treatment are too often uncertain and contingent upon individual patient variables. When it comes to the field of organizational behaviour, the biomedical model is even less well equipped to grasp the highly context-specific and uncertain factors that affect organizational and political change. The 'dialogue of the deaf' that results can be illustrated by the following peer reviewer comment in response to a draft article some of the authors prepared on the role of opinion leaders (since published, Locock et al. 2001). In response to the conclusion that it is difficult to interpret intervention studies of opinion leaders because locally contingent factors will affect their roles, the referee revealed the depth of difference and even plain bafflement between research paradigms:

I wonder if the authors would rethink [their] conclusion? . . . The idea of such local specificity with so much change between different places and the same place at different times suggests to me that the world is a more anarchic place than I can cope with.

As Strauss and Corbin (1990: 250) note, the usual scientific canon of reproducibility has limited value in real organizational circumstances:

Probably no theory that deals with a social/psychological phenomenon is actually reproducible, insofar as finding new situations or other situations whose conditions exactly match those of the original study, though many major conditions may be similar. Unlike the study of a physical phenomenon, it is very difficult to set up experimental or other designs in which one can re-create all of the original conditions and control all of the extraneous variables that may impinge upon the social/psychological phenomenon under investigation.

3.6   From EBHC to EBP?

EBHC has exerted considerable influence, and its apparent success has prompted many other policy areas to seek to follow suit. Three extremely helpful reviews of EBP in other sectors include Davies et al. (2000), a special edition of *Public Money and Management* (Davies et al. 1999), and Trinder and Reynolds (2000). As Klein (2000: 65) argues:

The notion is as seductive as it is simple: if evidence-based medicine is desirable then so, by definition, is evidence-based policy. Just as no one would argue that clinicians should practise medicine without regard to evidence, so it would seem an incontestable, self-evident proposition.

However, he argues that EBP is in fact 'highly contestable and mis-guided', for two linked reasons. One reason is that even within EBHC, as we have discussed within this chapter, the notion of evidence is more contested than it appears at first sight. If scientific certainty is elusive even in the world of clinical interventions, then a fortiori the problems become far worse in other evidence-based movements where research evidence is so much more ambiguous and contingent.

The second reason is that the idea of EBP 'rests on a gross misunderstanding of the policy process'; the policy process is in fact already driven by evidence, but of a very different kind from the narrow scientific view of evidence. Policy decisions incorporate evidence as to whether a policy will be implementable in practice, and whether it will be politically acceptable. Any policy that cannot meet this criteria is not worth pursuing, whatever the research evidence says.

A similar argument is made in a 1999 issue of *Public Money and Management* on the theme of evidence-based movements. The editors note striking differences between the acceptance of the need for evidence in health care and the view in other areas that 'the very nature of evidence is hotly disputed and there is strong resistance to assigning privileged status to one research method over another' (Davies et al. 1999). Research evidence has been only one ingredient in the policy process alongside, for example, ideology, professional and bureaucratic preferences, and public demand.

3.7   Concluding remarks

In this chapter, we have outlined the origins and rise of EBHC, and explored some of the reactions to it, notably amongst doctors themselves, managers, and policy-makers. The biomedical scientific base of EBHC has been one of its major strengths in appealing to the medical profession, and the history of EBM and latterly EBHC is characterized by strong professional leadership. Given medicine's continued autonomy and power to resist unwanted policy initiatives, it seems unlikely that EBHC would have got as far as it has without this professional support.

Amongst other evidence-based movements, EBP may be perceived more readily by practitioners as a managerially led means of control or cost-cutting, or an inappropriately reductionist view of what matters in policy decisions. Other professions may, of course, have less power than medicine to subvert or to reject EBPs they do not agree with, but the difficulties of imposing change in the face of resistance should not be underestimated. There are important lessons to learn from the history of EBHC about professional reactions to an evidence-based approach and the need to ensure professional ownership. How this is achieved will vary from profession to profession, but must take into account existing values, practices, and beliefs about both the nature and the provenance of what constitutes legitimate evidence.

The next chapter seeks to document our various research activities exploring the implication of EBHC within the setting of the English NHS. Specifically, we describe the research that we draw on in exploring the upscaling of qualitative research and reflect on the process we went through.

4

Research Design: 'Upscaling' Qualitative Research

Louise Locock, Ewan Ferlie, Sue Dopson, and Louise Fitzgerald

4.1 Introduction

Academic disciplines often display distinctive research paradigms, which in turn reflect their different basic assumptions about the nature of knowledge. These research paradigms need to be surfaced and discussed so that any paradigmatic choices made can be explicitly recognized and their implications for research design and method debated. A research paradigm provides an integrated set of assumptions about the nature of knowledge upon which the formulation of specific research questions and the adoption of particular research techniques are based. Patton (1978: 203, quoted in Oakley 2001: 27) indicates the potential deep power of a 'taken-for-granted' research paradigm:

[P]aradigms are deeply embedded in the socialisation of adherents and practitioners; paradigms tell them what is important, legitimate and reasonable. Paradigms are also normative, telling the practitioner what to do.

The concept of a research paradigm was famously proposed by Kuhn (1962) in his analysis of the evolution of scientific knowledge. Kuhn characterized a mature branch of science as having an accepted paradigm in which most research within that discipline would be done. In the early stages, there may be many schools of thought, but eventually one paradigm becomes dominant. The existing paradigm lasts until anomalies that it cannot explain accumulate and are championed. The field then enters into a rare period of 'revolutionary science' (or paradigm shift) where competing paradigms are in contest, out of which one becomes dominant in turn—not necessarily because it is any more valid than the old paradigm, but because it proves more useful to the scientific community at that point. Kuhn argues that each paradigm embodies such different assumptions that a gestalt switch in perception is needed to move from one to another (such as the shift from Newtonian to Einsteinian models in early twentieth-century physics). Such competing paradigms 'are not only incompatible but incommensurable' (Kuhn 1970: 103), so that the proponents of differ-ent paradigms 'argue past each other', employing different assump-tions, language, and technique (this argument was applied to the discipline of organizational sociology itself by Burrell and Morgan 1979).

Such processes can easily lead to so-called 'paradigm wars' (Oakley 2001) between different groups of researchers and associated discip-lines that are collocated within the same research field. Oakley (2001) suggests that the (contested) growth of qualitative social science over the last thirty or so years has had the effect of igniting paradigm wars in a number of fields where the social and natural sciences are collo-cated, including health services research (HSR). She warns against the crude negative stereotyping sometimes apparent between adherents of the two paradigms, and enjoins them to consider how they might possibly complement each other. There is an increasing number of multidisciplinary research teams, for instance, which are seeking to bring together the insights of different disciplines when working on a complex, multifaceted problem.

This chapter considers issues of research paradigms and associated methods of HSR. We seek here to reflect on the interpretive paradigm and in particular on the signs of rigour within qualitative research. The bulk of the chapter presents the nature of our work together and details of the seven studies that are used in the subsequent chapters of this book.

4.2   The positivistic paradigm and HSR

In Chapter 2 we reflected on some of the issues confronting those restudying complex organizations in health care. We noted in general that within the broad field of HSR, we can distinguish between two basic research paradigms: the positivistic paradigm (located in its biomedical and economics heartland) and the interpretive paradigm (strong in sociological, organizational, and anthropological studies). HSR grew up within the sphere of biomedical research, although there has recently been significant broadening with the growth of research into service delivery and organizational issues (Fulop et al. 2001). Within this arena, a wider range of non-traditional forms of research methods (e.g. action research) is evident than in other fields of HSR.

Within the positivistic HSR paradigm, an explicit 'hierarchy-of-evidence model' (Deek *et al.* 1996; Phase 5) has been developed, which is used to accord the different studies uncovered in a systematic literature review an 'appropriate weight' in the stage of synthesis. It is argued that this hierarchy reflects the extent to which the different designs ordered within it may be subject to bias. The well-designed randomized control trial (RCT) stands at the apex of this hierarchy of evidence (Table 4.1) and should in this view carry most weight in synthesis, at least where this type of RCT-based evidence is available to the reviewer. There is here considerable doubt about the validity of statistically combining the results of studies with different designs (cross-design synthesis) or synthesizing results of observational or uncontrolled studies, as this may lead to bias (Deek et al. 1996: Phase 5).

This research style has been reinforced by the rapid growth of the Cochrane Centre and associated collaborations in the late 1990s, which typically seek to collect and synthesize RCT-based evidence in particular sectors (see Chapter 3). However, the use of quasi-experimentalist designs within social science has also been critiqued by a number of prominent researchers. Within the field of criminological evaluation, for example, Pawson and Tilley (1997) see it as methodologically

Table 4.1 *An example of a hierarchy of evidence*

I	Well-designed randomized controlled trials
Other types of trial	
II-1a	Well-designed controlled trials with pseudo-randomization
II-1b	Well-designed controlled trials with no randomization
Cohort studies	
II-2a	Well-designed cohort (prospective study) with concurrent controls
II-2b	Well-designed cohort (prospective study) with historical controls
II-2c	Well-designed cohort (retrospective study) with concurrent controls
II-3	Well-designed case control (retrospective) study
III	Large differences in comparisons between times and places with or without intervention (in some circumstances these may be equivalent to Level II or I)
IV	Opinions of respected authorities based on clinical experience, descriptive studies, and reports of expert committees

Source: Deeks et al. 1996: 5.1

inappropriate. For example, it ignores the task of building theory, which can provide important explanation of the cause-and-effect relationships empirically detected within the quasi-experiment. Their own model of so-called 'realistic evaluation' portrays causation in the following terms: mechanism plus context equals outcome; that is,

> outcomes are explained by the action of particular mechanisms in particular contexts and this explanatory structure is put in place over time by a combination of theory and experimental observation. (Pawson and Tilley 1997: 59)

Note here the stress on 'why', 'how', and 'what' questions, which requires the development of an explanatory theoretical framework as well as empirical observation. The question of whether social theory is an important form of explanation (as we would agree) or an academic indulgence represents one controversy between advocates of quasi-experiments and realistic evaluation. We add that intermediate processes are important as are final outcomes, and indeed the quality of the process may help shape outcomes. Pawson and Tilley's model also draws attention to the mediating role of context in shaping outcomes. An appreciation of context cannot then be factored out as a residual through randomization; rather it has to be an integral part of the explanation.

4.3   The interpretive paradigm and HSR

The interpretive paradigm within HSR is associated with certain social sciences, such as medical sociology, anthropology, and organizational studies. Organizational and management studies have grown rapidly as a field of teaching and research over the last thirty or so years, as evident in the MBA boom but also in the emergence of a fundamental research base and high-quality journals in which research is published (Ferlie et al. 2001). There is increased interest in organizational and management research in the health sector, as in other sectors.

The interpretive paradigm is interested in the study of meanings that social actors attach to their actions, for example what shapes the pattern of interactions between doctors and patients. It would be interested in how we can describe the organizational culture (or various subcultures) of a health care organization. It is also more interested in understanding subjective experience than 'objective' data, and would argue that such numerical data are themselves often the product of processes of social construction (e.g. there may be a tendency for deaths from stigmatized causes such as suicide or HIV/ AIDS to be under-recorded on death certificates, due to a protective social relationship between the recording doctor and relatives). Interpretive methods are particularly indicated where the task is the description, interpretation, and explanation of a phenomenon rather than estimation of its prevalence (Lee 1999).

Within the interpretive camp, there is a division of opinion between radical social constructivists on the one hand and 'critical realists' on the other. Critical realists accept that 'things happen' (as in Pawson and Tilley's model of realistic evaluation, which indeed deals with 'real' social phenomena such as car theft) but that different stakeholder groups may have a range of interpretations of their significance that need to be incorporated within analysis.

However, all interpretivists would be likely to argue that there are severe limitations in the applicability of quasi-experimental methods to the exploration of social phenomena: studying people is not like studying molecules. Critics argue that the quasi-experimental model has promised much but produced little in the field of public policy research (Pawson and Tilley 1997). The quasi-experimental model is held to be particularly inappropriate in the investigation of broad or diffuse problems; in problems that involve important social relationships (indeed branches of medicine that are more socially orientated, such as primary care, experience greater difficulties in applying a 'pure' RCT research model and display more non-experimental research methods); and where the researcher has a low level of control over the setting.

Organizational studies is one important strand within interpretive approaches to HSR, along with other disciplines such as anthropology and medical sociology. As indicated in Chapter 2, the main intellectual trend here (at least in the UK) has been a drift from positivistic and functionalist methods (which, firstly, assume that organizational structures can be measured and, secondly, that these structures reflect in a relatively non-problematic manner the impact of forces from the environment) to more interpretive approaches, including feminist, action research, and postmodernist forms of analysis (Clegg et al. 1996). Calas and Smirnich (1999) argue that the increased questioning of postmodern writers has led to alternative methods and allowed new 'voices' to be heard in organizational studies. Much UK organizational research is presently of a qualitative nature.

4.4   What are the signs of rigour within qualitative research?

We now move from a discussion of alternative research paradigms to an exploration of what might be considered good quality research within each paradigm, especially the interpretive paradigm. The positivistic paradigm already utilizes a hierarchy-of-evidence model, which enables researchers to distinguish between different grades of evidence. The question of what might constitute parallel indicators of 'rigour' within qualitative research into health care organizations is more complex and it is not possible to produce an analogous hierarchy-of-evidence model within qualitative research (Deek et al. 2001). But the question 'What does good qualitative research look like?' is an increasingly important one (compare the much greater attention paid to the assessment of qualitative research in Deek et al. 2001 than Deek et al. 1996). Clearly it is possible to produce bad qualitative research, such as where there is no research protocol at all (Yin 1999). Some qualitative HSR researchers are developing alternative indicators of quality (Murphy et al. 1998; Yin 1999), although this process is still in its early stages. Mays et al. (2001) compared the assessment frameworks developed by three qualitative HSR groups (Blaxter 1996; Mays and Pope 2000; Popay et al. 1998). All three groups suggested the following criteria of quality:

- consideration of the appropriateness of the methods used for the question and subject matter and why qualitative methods were appropriate;
- adequacy of sampling, which is as much an issue in qualitative as quantitative research, and clear explanation of the sampling strategy;
- the rigour of data analysis—was it conducted in a systematic way? Does it succeed in incorporating all the observations and dealing with variation?
- the reflexivity of the account—'sensitivity to the ways in which the researcher and research process have shaped the data collected' (Mays and Pope 2000: 96) and the provision of sufficient information about the research process to enable readers to judge this;
- adequacy of presentation of findings—is it clear how the analysis flows from the data? Is sufficient data presented to justify conclusions?
- worth and relevance of that research.

4.5   Case study design

In this book we are specifically concerned with qualitative research based on case studies, and it is worth pausing to reflect on the nature and value of the case study. There are many texts discussing the case study method. Perhaps the most widely cited is Yin's *Case Study Research: Design and Methods*. According to him, the case study seeks to explore a contemporary phenomenon within a real life context, where the phenomenon and the context are not clearly evident, and in which multiple sources of evidence are used (Yin 1994: 23).

The most frequently encountered definitions of case studies have usually repeated the types of topic to which case studies have been applied, for example:

[T]he essence of a case study, the central tendency among all types of case study, is that it tries to illuminate a decision or set of decisions: why they were taken, how they were implemented and with what result. (Schramm 1997)

Case studies also have a distinctive place in evaluation research (Patton 1980). They can help explain the causal links in real-life interventions that are too complex for the survey or experimental strategies; describe the 'real-life' context in which an intervention has occurred; provide an illustrative description of the intervention itself; and explore those situations in which the intervention being evaluated has no clear, single set of outcomes.

Another important difference within case study research is the extent to which a longitudinal perspective is taken, where researchers purposefully seek to take account of the impact of 'history' on the present. Longitudinal case studies, developed over many months or years, will produce a richer form of data that differs from cross-sectional snapshot studies, where the data are collected in one short burst, over several weeks. Data collected in real time may vary from retrospective data, where the respondents will have reflected on events and their, now known, consequences, and where they may also have forgotten some nuances of what occurred. Within process research, a sustained period of real-time data collection is likely to be the strongest method, if that is practically feasible.

4.5.1   *Improving the quality of case study research*

Fulfilling the promise of case studies, as well as contributing to theory and policy development, requires researchers to meet some important standards for good quality case study research. One of the contributing authors of this book (Ferlie 2002) recently suggested candidate domains of research quality within qualitative health care management research, which include:

- *research relevance*, an area in which research engages with broad public policy or concern, giving voice to excluded groups and contributing to positive social and organizational change;
- *reliability*, defined in terms of whether there is an audit trail that would, in principle, allow another researcher to replicate the study so that an investigator who repeated the investigation and reran the same case study would obtain the same results (as argued by Yin 1994);
- *internal validity* (does the account accurately and deeply portray the social and organizational settings studied?) and *external validity* (are these findings of wider significance beyond the immediate setting?) are important in the assessment of qualitative health care management research. A good quality case study should certainly offer high internal validity when compared to alternative strategies of investigation such as social surveys. The reader will still need to be reassured about the extent to which the investigator has been immersed in the field, the approach to sampling taken, and whether all key stakeholders have been accessed.

  Achieving higher levels of external validity may be more problematic, as some evidence from an audit of key journals (Ferlie 2002) indicates that UK health management research is characterized by the production of the single case from which it is difficult to generalize and which is largely non-cumulative in nature. Responses to this weakness designed to ensure a greater level of external validity include larger scale and comparative case designs; purposeful replication of major earlier studies; benchmarking against related studies within the literature; and greater conceptual generalization to theory;
- *construct validity* (Yin 1994) draws attention to the quality of middle-range theory and concept building within qualitative research. It suggests the importance of careful theory operationalization (from theory to the field) and reconnection (from data to theory) so that the themes or processes studied are clearly related to an operationalized theory. An example would be to specify how the relatively loose concept of *context* might affect change processes and why.

Yin (1999) has also recently discussed how the methodological quality of case studies within HSR might be improved. He noted that the difficulty of generalizing from cases has been seen as a major short-coming of the method (a low level of external validity). One way in which external validity can be increased is through theory-building. Yin argues that each case study, as a unit, can be considered a single experiment: a multiple case study can be considered as multiple experiments. Yin suggests that an appropriate response to the need to build external validity through theory is not to select cases through a sampling logic, but through a replication logic:

[T]he needed replication logic can be derived only from hypotheses or theories about the cases. In other words, a theory about what is being studied—and about whether a single case is a 'critical' exemplar of that theory or about why some multiple cases might be expected to be replications and others might not—is essential to case study design and analysis. (Yin 1999: 1213)

Flyvbjerg (2001) explains how a single 'critical' case study can in itself lead to generalization through falsification. Taking Karl Popper's famous example of 'all swans are white', which would be falsified by a single observation of a black swan, Flyvbjerg (2001: 77) suggests:

[T]he case study is well-suited to identifying 'black swans' because of its in-depth approach: what appears to be 'white' often turns out on closer examination to be 'black'.

At the same time, however, Flyvbjerg argues that attempts by social science to emulate natural science—'physics envy'—are fundamentally misplaced, and that 'formal generalization is overvalued'. This is a question we return to below.

Eisenhardt (1989) highlights a lack of clarity about the process of building theory from multiple cases, especially regarding the central inductive process and the role of the literature. She acknowledges the work on grounded theory-building by Glaser and Strauss (1967) and Miles and Huberman's work (1984) outlining techniques for analysing qualitative data in seeking to present in her article a 'more nearly complete roadmap' for executing case study research. In her view strong case studies 'are those which present interesting or frame-breaking theories which meet the tests of good theory or concept development (e.g. parsimony, testability, logical influence) and are grounded in convincing evidence' (Eisenhardt 1989: 549). Health care studies in the UK have been criticized for a lack of theoretical grounding and deemed not to meet such tests (Stewart 1999: 2).

4.6   Upscaling: a search for higher external validity

The question of generalization provokes radically different responses amongst social scientists. Flyvbjerg's concern that generalization is overvalued was noted in the preceding section, although this does not mean he precludes generalization altogether. Indeed he states that it can be appropriate and valuable in some cases, but is at pains to stress that it is not the only way to work. He also argues that despite the difficulties of summarizing qualitative research, case studies can still contribute to cumulative development of knowledge, not least through hypothesis testing and falsification, which is possible from single cases, let alone multiple cases. Nonetheless, he concludes that

if we want to recover social science from its current role as loser in the Science Wars . . . we must drop the fruitless efforts to emulate natural science's success in producing cumulative and predictive theory. (Flyvbjerg 2001: 116)

The extreme radical social constructionist position is that generalization is neither desirable nor feasible. Campbell et al. (2003: 683), for example, note that

synthesising qualitative research is a contentious issue for the qualitative research community because it rests on a number of contested assumptions about the nature and purpose of qualitative research. In particular, it presupposes that it is reasonable to generalise beyond individual qualitative studies. Postmodernists reject outright any form of generalisation and so will not regard qualitative research synthesis as a legitimate approach. Others, although not rejecting generalisation altogether will be concerned that in synthesising across different studies important differences will be downplayed and that the real value of qualitative research, in terms of its emphasis on context and holism, will be lost.

Even the authors of one of the central texts on qualitative synthesis or 'meta-ethnography', Noblit and Hare (1988), make no claim to generalization on the basis of a comparative approach to case studies. Whilst positivists see accumulation of knowledge as a means to develop predictions, 'anticipation, rather than prediction, is the more reasonable result of qualitative research'. An accumulation of qualitative studies in a particular field may simply reflect the fact that it is an enduring area of concern—'it may or may not reflect a substantive improvement in how well we understand something' (Noblit and Hare 1988: 25).

However, Noblit and Hare are concerned with theory development. In their own field of educational research, they suggest that the quality of individual studies is high, but efforts to be highly grounded and empirical have led to relative neglect of 'the theoretical and philosophical issues that enable the paradigm to flourish and grow. If the paradigm seeks to create a knowledge base and inform practice, then we must find ways to synthesise our research' (Noblit and Hare 1988: 23).

They develop what they call a 'line-of-argument' approach as the key contribution of qualitative synthesis, which is 'essentially about inference—what can we say of the whole . . . based on selective studies of the parts? This is the same as basic theorising in qualitative research'. In this sense, as Geertz (1973: 26) argues, theory is used 'to ferret out the unapparent import of things' or, as Noblit and Hare (1988: 75) describe it, 'to reveal what is hidden in individual studies'. Initial levels of synthesis help elucidate similarities and differences between studies, whereas line-of-argument synthesis 'goes one step further and puts any similarities and differences into a new interpretive context. In short the translation of cases into one another sets the stage for a second-level inference about the relationship between the studies'. Unlike quantitative meta-analysis, the aim of qualitative synthesis is to be interpretive rather than aggregative—the raw material of meta-analysis is numerical data, which can be added together, whereas the raw material of qualitative synthesis is interpretations, which are then subjected to another layer of interpretation or 'reciprocal translation'.

The concern with synthesis as a means of theoretical advancement rather than as a positivist means of accumulating generalizable 'facts' is echoed in Pawson's conception of 'realist synthesis' (Pawson 2002). This extends earlier work using a realist interpretive approach to programme evaluation (Pawson and Tilley 1997). Pawson also identifies falsification as a key component of case study research, with the added assertion that understanding where and why a particular innovation fails, we can also glean 'vital clues on when and how it can succeed' (Pawson 2002: 346). This is not falsification by individual researchers seeking to prove their own hypotheses wrong. Rather, 'cumulation of understanding occurs across the body of research and so it occurs collectively as the second researcher tries to correct the errors of the first'.

The way in which evidence is assembled together to reveal the policy lesson exposes, however, crucial differences between the aims and content of various types of synthesis. Pawson distinguishes three broad categories:

1. *Meta-analysis* searches for reliable measures (preferably through RCTs) of the net effect of different programmes, performing calculations to reveal 'best-buy' programmes. This views programmes as exercising a straightforward causal effect (a 'successionist' view of causation).

2. *Narrative review* takes a 'configurational' view of causality, namely that 'outcomes are considered to follow from the alignment of a fruitful combination of attributes' (Pawson 2002: 341). Rather than producing a generalizable 'best buy', narrative review identifies successful 'exemplary cases' and proposes that those seeking to imitate the programme should try as far as possible to recreate those favourable circumstances, or as many of them as possible.

3. *Realist synthesis*, as with realistic evaluation, takes a 'generative' approach to causation. It is not 'programmes' that work, but the 'underlying reasons or resources' (Pawson 2002: 342) they offer to participants that generate change. Furthermore, outcomes are contingent upon the context: both the nature of the participants and the circumstances of the site. The question is 'what works for whom and in what circumstances', and the result is therefore not a 'best-buy' universal programme recommendation. Instead, 'realist synthesis delves into inconsistencies to build "programme theories"'' (Pawson 2002: 346).

Thus Pawson (2002: 347) argues that

the basic idea of systematic review is to draw transferable lessons from existing programmes and initiatives. Realist synthesis assumes that the transmission of lessons occurs through a process of theory-building rather than assembling empirical generalisations.

Others working within an interpretive paradigm adopt a similar position on the importance of context in determining what we can extract in the way of generalization. Noblit and Hare (1988), for example, note the tendency of quantitative synthesis to ignore 'meaning in context' because it is seen to get in the way of producing generalizable findings. It is treated as a confounding variable that must be controlled, or stripped out of the equation, rather than understood as an important explanatory variable. Context-stripping may help focus on commonalities and assist in the production of a short synthesis, but it impedes proper interpretive synthesis.

Ragin has been developing the idea of qualitative comparative analysis, a new analytic technique that uses Boolean algebra to facilitate multiple comparisons of case studies and identify patterns of configurations of factors which lead to particular outcomes. Ragin (2000: 15) suggests:

[T]he main contrast is between the conventional view of causation as a context between individual variables to explain variation in an outcome and the diversity-oriented view that causality is both conjectural and multiple. In the conventional view, each single causal condition, conceived as an analytically distinct variable, has an independent impact on the outcome. In the diversity-oriented view, causes combine in different and sometimes contradictory ways to produce the same outcome, revealing different paths.

Ragin is interested to explain how the same outcome can be arrived at in different ways, and to identify through comparative studies the number and character of different causal models that can account for this same outcome. One might add that exploration of different causal models accounting for *different* outcomes is an equally valuable exercise, and one closer to Pawson's identification of patterns of positive and negative outcomes from the same programme in varying contexts.

Flyvbjerg (2001) devotes an entire chapter to the fact that 'context matters', although he takes a more radical view in concluding that social science faces an irresolvable paradox. Context is central for understanding human action and indeed for understanding what counts as an action from the actors' point of view. There are no universal laws or rules by which we can predict human behaviour. Yet 'context must nevertheless be excluded in a theory in order for it to be a theory at all' (Flyvbjerg 2001: 42), in the sense that theory is by definition understood as predictive and explanatory. 'It is this contradiction which punctures the aspirations of the social sciences to become normal sciences' (Flyvbjerg 2001: 42).

As the above discussion begins to suggest, not only is there debate about what are feasible goals for qualitative synthesis, and the extent to which generalization and cumulation are possible, but there is also a welter of different terms and techniques in use. There is no doubt that it is attracting increased academic interest, stimulated (certainly in HSR) at least partly by the development of quantitative meta-analysis. In addition to the term 'qualitative synthesis' we have already encountered above the terms 'meta-ethnography', 'narrative review', and 'realist synthesis'. 'Narrative (meta)-synthesis', 'meta-synthesis', 'qualitative systematic review', 'data synthesis of qualitative research' and doubtless many other terms abound in what has been aptly described as a 'lexiconic mess'!

The background of developments in quantitative meta-analysis and systematic review is important for understanding some manifestations of the interest in synthesizing qualitative research. For example, a search on the terms 'qualitative' and 'systematic' on the MEDLINE, EMBASE, and CINAHL databases yields many studies that are undertaking 'qualitative systematic review'. However, the meaning of this seems, in many cases, to be identical to 'systematic review', which is only qualitative in the sense that it is combining text-based reports of RCT findings, rather than full numerical aggregation as would be the case in meta-analysis. For example, Campbell et al. (2001) have published an article reporting a qualitative systematic review of whether cannabinds are an effective and safe treatment option for pain management. The design is 'a systematic review of randomised controlled trials'. Twenty were identified, of which eleven were excluded. Outcomes examined were pain intensity scores, pain relief scores, and adverse effects. This is, of course, a valuable exercise, but is not relevant for any consideration of synthesizing primarily qualitative studies.

A further category of interest is articles that are keen to see more formal inclusion of qualitative evidence in systematic reviews, alongside RCT and other experimental data. An example would be the examination of current practice and methodological challenges by Dixon-Woods et al. (2001). The National Health Service Centre for Reviews and Dissemination (Deek et al. 1996) guidelines for undertaking systematic reviews of research on effectiveness also argues that 'qualitative research involving comparison between sites and cases can increase confidence in the generality of a finding or explanation' (Kahn et al. 2001: 20), and suggest the work of Noblit and Hare (1988) as a possible methodological guide, although it is noted that the development of formal procedures for 'narrative synthesis' has received little attention so far.

The Economic and Social Research Council (ESRC) has commissioned a two-year study precisely to address this question (www.ccsr.ac.uk/methods/projects/posters/popay.shtml). The research outline notes:

Statistical approaches to combining findings from different studies in systematic reviews of evidence are well developed. However, these techniques are not always appropriate. Narrative approaches to evidence synthesis are therefore being developed but these do not rest on an authoritative body of knowledge. This project will develop, test and disseminate methodological guidance on 'good practice' in narrative synthesis.

Although these sources are careful to allow for qualitative research as 'a methodologically sufficient approach in its own right' (Dixon-Woods et al. 2001: 125), the particular interest here is how qualitative research can add to and elucidate quantitative systematic reviews. For example, the research objectives for the ESRC programme include:

- to review the methodological literature on narrative approaches to evidence synthesis;
- to assess existing approaches to narrative synthesis in a sample of systematic reviews;
- to produce draft guidance on best practice for the narrative synthesis of quantitative and qualitative data.

Guidance on narrative synthesis in systematic reviews will be included in Cochrane and Campbell Reviewers Handbooks and the next iteration of the Deek et al. 1996 guidelines for Undertaking Systematic Reviews (Kahn et al. 2001).

Again, this is an entirely acceptable aim, but it tends in this instance to characterize qualitative research as a helpful adjunct to systematic reviews. Narrative in this sense is more about using words to provide a bridge between quantitative and qualitative research on similar topics. In Pawson's terms, one might argue that this remains more about 'assembling empirical generalisations' from multiple studies (Pawson 2002: 347), rather than the interpretive, theory-building exercise he and Noblit and Hare (1988) would advocate.

Finally there are those who are debating and experimenting with qualitative meta-synthesis and meta-ethnography as an exercise in its own right. Although Noblit and Hare come from an educational research background, much of the interest in their techniques has come from nursing studies, for example, the volume by Paterson et al. (2001) in *Sage's Methods in Nursing Research Series*. This discusses the theory and techniques of meta-synthesis and also uses practical examples drawn from the author's experience of meta-study of qualitative research on chronic illness.

Sandelowski (1997: 367) identify three kinds of qualitative meta-synthesis:

1. The integration of findings from individual pieces of research carried out by the same investigator (e.g. the work of Rogers

1995, or the work of a team of investigators led by a single director in the case of Van de Ven 1992).

2. The synthesis of findings across studies carried out by different investigators (used by Sandelowski herself in a recent article, Sandelowski and Barroso 2003).

3. The use of quantitative methods to aggregate qualitative findings (e.g. the case survey method, using highly structured questions to collect information from separate case studies on a particular theme, which can then be turned into a data-set for statistical analysis).

Campbell et al. (2003) report their own experience of using Noblit and Hare's meta-ethnography framework to synthesize seven studies of lay experience of diabetes and diabetes care and how they feel this contrasts with conventional quantitative meta-analysis. Whereas meta-analysis is 'concerned with aggregating data in order to have sufficient statistical power to detect a cause-and-effect relationship between a particular treatment and specific health outcomes', the synthesis of qualitative research

can be envisaged as the bringing together of findings on a chosen theme, the results of which should, in conceptual terms, be greater than the sum of parts. Thus, the purpose of a qualitative synthesis would be to achieve greater understanding and attain a level of conceptual or theoretical development beyond that achieved in any individual empirical study. This implies that qualitative synthesis would go beyond the description and summarising associated with a narrative literature review and be quite distinct from a quantitative meta-analysis in that it would not entail the simple aggregation of findings. Like a secondary analysis, qualitative synthesis could involve reinterpretation, but unlike secondary analysis it would be based on published findings rather than primary data. (Campbell et al. 2003: 672)

The process of 'reciprocal translation' to examine key concepts across the studies is similar to the process of constant comparison used in qualitative analysis of primary data, which leads to the development of second-order constructs; in meta-ethnography, this moves a stage further to develop third-order constructs from second-order data. These new synthesized concepts may not have been explicitly identified in any of the original empirical studies under review. This is an example of a 'line-of-argument synthesis': the construction of an interpretation which, as Campbell et al. (2003: 680) summarize it, 'serves to reveal what is hidden in individual studies and to discover a whole among a set of parts'. For example, they identify the notion of 'strategic non-compliance' as part of the lay experience of diabetes. This was common to, but not previously explicit in, the studies synthesized. (Strategic non-compliance is defined as the thoughtful and selective application of medical advice, rather than blind adherence to it, which in turn gives a greater sense of control and coping.)

Campbell et al. acknowledge concerns in some postmodernist quarters that generalization from individual qualitative accounts is simply not legitimate. They conclude that 'synthesising qualitative research does not replace the need for individual studies', but argue that it can add to the findings in the originals. They characterize meta-ethnography as 'an interpretive endeavour, the purpose of which is to achieve a greater degree of conceptual development and insight than was attained in the original individual studies' (Campbell et al. 2003: 683). They note that none of the six studies published after the first one included in their synthesis made any reference to each other's work, and that, therefore, none had built upon previous findings in this field or attempted to compare findings.

4.7 Our methods

From what has been discussed so far, it is clear that a potentially important methodological contribution lies in 'scaling up' the low level of empirically founded external validity achieved in much current UK health management research (Ferlie 2002). A move from single to multiple case designs is one way of increasing external validity empirically. In this monograph, we are seeking to build an overview across a family of related studies drawing on our experience of research in this area. This cross-study perspective is different from an ethnographic approach to case-study-based research, which would stress the achievement of deep insight within a single case.

Our own work discussed below is a further attempt to 'scale up' qualitative and case-study-based empirical data and test how one can do this in a methodologically rigorous way. Although it has much in common with other attempts at synthesis described above, we would argue that it has certain distinctive features. The literature on qualitative synthesis tends to focus on the analysis of secondary, published data, often by researchers who were not involved in any of the original studies. Our own approach is perhaps a step further back in the chain, in that we are using our final research reports, which are much longer and more detailed than the findings presented in a peer-review article. Furthermore, we have the advantage of being able to go back to the primary data when needed (e.g. to check for further quotations) and we have the primary data in our shared memory. Indeed, the process of going back and forth between primary data, the final reports, and the synthesis have continued throughout the preparation of the book. As Noblit and Hare (1988: 24) anticipate, our experience has been that 'in the process of studying something, interpretivists often discover a new area of discourse. . . . An unanticipated understanding may develop that teaches us the limitations of the discourse we originally intended to inform'. As one pursues the original interest that sparked off the attempt at synthesis, 'what is of interest undoubtedly changes. It may be modified, specified or elaborated'.

Unlike the type of synthesis noted by Sandelowski (1997), which involves the integration of findings from individual pieces of research carried out by the same investigator, we have brought together two teams of investigators and pooled our separately conducted studies that we believe meet the tests of rigour in qualitative research discussed in Section 4.4. Finally there is the question of sheer scale—for example, Campbell et al. (2003) synthesize findings from seven studies comprising 193 interviews, and Sandelowski and Barroso (2003) use forty-five studies with a total sample number of 925. We have sought to synthesize via discussion and debate over some four years the findings of forty-nine individual case studies and 1,400 interviews.

4.7.1 *Cross-study comparison: are our seven studies similar or different?*

Clearly, a guiding principle is that one needs to pool like with like: cross-design synthesis is as difficult in qualitative as quantitative work. The greater the similarity, the more methodologically appropriate synthetic work becomes. Cross-study comparison is easiest where there is a purposefully designed and prospective replication of an earlier design. It is therefore encouraging that four of our present set of studies form two replicated 'pairs': the 'Warwick team' undertook an early study analysing evidence-based medicine (EBM) implementation in the acute sector (Wood et al. 1998); this was followed deliberately by a replication by the same team in the primary care sector (Fitzgerald et al. 1999). As far as the 'Oxford/Southampton team' is concerned, the Wales study (Locock et al. 1999) was conducted explicitly as a continuation of the evaluation methods used in the Promoting Action on Clinical Effectiveness (PACE) project (Dopson et al. 1999).

However, the other three studies did not take the form of purpose-designed replications and pose more complexity for what is a retrospective overview. What methodological guidance do we have in this situation? Yin (1999) notes that an increasingly common situation in case-study-based research is for cases to be undertaken by multiple teams, in order to meet the tight project deadlines often found in HSR. His advice is that such teams need to display a common orientation and training and to follow similar field protocols. Without such common features, it is impossible to be clear whether any differences found between the cases are 'real' or artefactual due to interteam differences. We discuss later the process we went through to achieve 'a common orientation'.

In many respects, there are, however, important similarities between the studies. The seven studies were all undertaken within the same national health care system (the UK NHS), at the same period, the 1990s, so that two very important aspects of context (time period and geographical/organizational setting) are held constant. They were also undertaken by two teams of researchers who displayed similar theoretical and disciplinary bases, that is, they shared an organizational behaviour (OB) perspective and concepts. Both groups used similar—though not identical—comparative case study designs (there are no single case studies in the set and the number of cases in any study varies from four to sixteen) rather than experimental, observational, or indeed postmodernist or action research methods. All studies focused on the organizational and group levels of analysis rather than single individuals. There was a common unit of analysis across the studies, namely a social analysis of the career of EBHC ideas and innovation in 'real-world' health care settings. The material generated and analysed in the studies was verbal and literary (rather than numeric) in nature, typically taking the form of case studies, which are compared and contrasted within the individual study, first of all to identify trends and tendencies. Cross-study pooling continues this comparative logic, which is already apparent in the individual studies. All the studies used documentary analyses and in-depth and semi-structured interviews as important data collection methods. The analysis strategy used in all cases was content analysis, and in one study NUDIST qualitative software was used.

Table 4.2 presents an overview of the research design and methods across the seven related studies undertaken by the two groups. Taken as a whole, we conclude that this represents a related family of studies, which share important core features so that cross-study pooling is methodologically appropriate.

There are some particular methodological problems in comparing the results from the studies listed in Table 4.2. The studies are similar but not identical in nature, and we need to be alert to these differences. Resource constraints help explain the decision to use telephone interviews rather than face-to-face interviews in four studies. Four studies used written questionnaires as part of data collection and three did not. Besides these relatively obvious differences, a number of deeper methodological challenges faced us in comparing results across the seven studies.

The process we have gone through has been an iterative one involving several stages; during and after each stage we reflected critically on the methodological experience and recorded our reflections. This was carried out both through collective discussion at meetings and individual written reflections that were shared with the rest of the group. The main stages are described below.

Stage 1: initial overview

We made a decision early on that we would use the final published reports of each research project as the basis for our work together (Dopson and Gabbay 1995; CSAG 1998; Dawson et al. 1998; Wood et al. 1998; Dopson et al. 1999; Fitzgerald et al. 1999; Locock et al. 1999). Given the number of interviews and case studies involved, we did not feel it was practical to go back to these original sources, although we did on occasions go back to the original data to assist clarification. The final reports alone contain approximately 200,000 words when added together.

At this first stage, every member of both research teams reread all the detailed final project reports. Additionally, each team produced a summary of what they felt were the key points arising from their own studies. An important point to note is that to some extent the final reports were already cumulative or comparative, given that each team was building on its past research and that both teams were already in communication with each other and citing each other's findings in some of the later reports. For example, reflections on the socially constructed nature of scientific research evidence and the existence of competing bodies of evidence formed a prominent part

Table 4.2 *An overview of the research design and methods across the seven sites*

	Design	No. of case studies	Face-to-face interviews*	Telephone interviews*	Written questionnaires	Document analysis	Dates
Dopson and Gabbay 1995	Single-stage case studies on four clinical topics	4	58 (RHA and purchasing managers, clinicians and public health)			√	2 years, 1993–4
Wood et al. 1998a	Two stages: 1. Overview survey across whole region		71 (mainly front-line clinicians)			√	2 years, 1995–7
	2. Case studies, one per clinical topic, selected on evidence of clinical change elicited from first stage	4	48 (mainly clinicians and clinical managers)			√	2 years, 1995–7
Dawson et al. 1998	Embedded case studies, two clinical topics in each of four hospitals	8	256 (clinical staff of various professions and grades) plus 20 informal interviews with trust and HA managers		256 (same group as interviews)	√	2 years, 1995–7
CSAG, 1998	Single-stage case study design, full in seven sites, telephone and questionnaire only in six	13 (7+6)	250 (front-line clinicians and managers)	321	1317 GPs, 256 hospital clinicians	√	6 months, 1996–7
Fitzgerald et al. 1999	Three stages: 1. Overview across four health authorities on diffusion of innovation		38 (senior HA managers and GPs)			√	2 years, 1997–9
	2. Overview with same		35				2 years, 1997–9

	group, concentrated on particular innovations						
	3. Case studies on four innovations in primary care	4	40 (GPs and other primary care and physiotherapy staff)			√	2 years, 1997–9
Dopson et al. 1999	Two stages: 1. Initial round of interviews half-way through project	16	7 (staff from King's Fund and DoH)	51 (project team members— managers and clinicians)		√	2 years, 1997–8
	2. Second round at end of project, using themes elicited during first stage			122 (project team members, other senior managers and clinicians)	150 (front-line clinicians)	√	2 years, 1997–8
Locock et al. 1999	Single-stage case studies, after project completion	6	18 (front-line clinicians)	65 (project team members, other senior managers and clinicians, Welsh Office reps)	238 (front-line clinicians)	√	6 months, 1998–9

* All interviews were in-depth and semi-structured.

of the Warwick acute study report (Wood et al. 1998), and influenced the Wales report (Locock et al. 1999). Meanwhile, the analysis by Dawson et al. (1998) of how the subjective understandings of clinicians mediate the flow of evidence into practice is cited in the Warwick primary care study (Fitzgerald et al. 1999).

From this stage we developed an initial overview of the findings, identifying common themes emerging from each team's separate key points. The major topics identified at this stage were:

- Evidence
- Context
- Professionals/opinion leaders

- Translation/interpretation
- Management/organization.

Stage 2:   pilot analysis of one theme by one researcher
As a pilot, one researcher undertook a more in-depth analysis of one theme (the impact of opinion leaders in encouraging or blocking clinical behaviour change), using the two sets of key points and the full text of the final reports. This was then commented on by other researchers, and we assessed the feasibility of pursuing this method for other themes. It was decided that for the next stage each researcher should undertake their own analysis of each theme to avoid reliance on one researcher's perceptions. At this stage, we also prepared an exploratory paper for the Organizational Behaviour in Healthcare Conference in Keele, January 2000 (since published as Ferlie et al. 2001), summarizing our experience to date and incorporating the overview of opinion leaders.

Stage 3:   analysis of one theme by all researchers
To support the next stage systematically, we prepared a draft coding structure of themes and sub-headings, which each team member then applied to the theme of the nature of the research evidence, working independently. Table 4.3 provides an extract from the draft coding structure relating to this theme, for illustration.

   This was followed by a collective discussion and simultaneous analysis using one report as an illustration. At this point, the draft coding categories were debated between all team members to check for perceived accuracy and completeness, and redrafted. Our work up to this point formed the basis for participation in a health care research symposium at the American Academy of Management in 2001 (since published as Dopson et al. 2002), and plans to work on a book were agreed.

Stage 4:   analysis of all themes by all researchers
At the next stage, each researcher individually applied the whole coding structure to all the themes and all the reports, looking for points of difference as well as convergence, and reflecting on (*a*) use of different terms to define similar areas and (*b*) use of similar terms but meaning different things. For example, we found uncertainties about definitions of product champions versus opinion leaders between teams (see further discussion below), and found differing layers of understanding of what we meant by 'context'. Again, the

Table 4.3   *Extract from draft coding structure*

Hierarchies of research evidence
- Differential acceptance by professional groups
- Different sources with greater or lesser credibility/authority

Availability/accessibility of sources of evidence
- Existence or otherwise of 'good' sources (libraries, CRD, etc.)
- How far were there sources for raw evidence or summaries/reviews?
- Skills needed to access them
- Equipment needed to access them
- Presence or absence of effective national and local dissemination strategies

'Strength' of evidence
- What is regarded as strong by different groups?
- Is it necessary to achieve change?
- Is it sufficient to achieve change?
- Strong evidence may be strong evidence that does not support change
- Strong evidence may not tell you *how* best to organize care

Weaker evidence
- Less likely to achieve change?
- How is weak evidence or gaps in evidence handled?

Other kinds of 'evidence'
- Experience/tacit knowledge
- Early training
- Continuing development training
- Expert opinion
- Peer opinion
- Norms of practice (local, national)
- Existing guidelines
- Royal colleges
- Patient views
- Awareness of other reasons to change, e.g. poor quality, need to save money, need to make processes more efficient
- Others?

---

outputs generated by all five researchers were debated collectively and aggregated. As this stage proceeded, a revised set of themes began to crystallize, and we developed a table (Table 4.4) assessing the comparative strength and importance of these themes in each study.

The approach we have piloted cannot be described as a systematic review or a meta-analysis in any formal sense, although it has some elements in common with those approaches and goes beyond the usual limited focus on one project. A more accurate characterization

Table 4.4   *Revised themes: comparative strength and importance*

Theme	Dopson and Gabbay 1995	Wood et al. 1998	Dawson et al. 1998	CSAG 1998	Fitzger- ald et al. 1999	Dopson et al. 1999	Locock et al. 1999
Evidence is not sufficient	3	2	3	3	3	3	3
Evidence is socially con- structed	2	3	3	2	3	3	3
Evidence is differentially available	2	3	2	3	3	1	2
Hierarchies of evidence exist	3	3	3	3	2	3	3
Other sources of evidence	2	2	3	3	3	2	3
The importance of professional networks	2	3	3	3	3	3	3
The role of professional boundaries	2	3	3	3	3	2	2
Context as an influence	3	2	3	3	3	3	3
The role of opinion leaders	2	2	3	3	3	3	3
The enactment of evidence	3	3	3	3	3	3	3

Key: 1 = theme is present; 2 = strong evidence of theme; 3 = very strong evidence of presence.

draws on the familiar technique in qualitative data analysis of pattern detection through constant comparison, but on a 'grand' scale. Pattern detection was of course an essential element of each separate research project; the research teams looked for patterns both amongst respondents within each case study and then across the case studies in each piece of research. Our subsequent synthesis experiment has essentially continued this process across the final reports of each research project, and the result is somewhere between the second-order and third-order constructs noted by Campbell et al. (2003).

4.8 Methodological challenges in cross-study synthesis

4.8.1 *The complexity of process data*

As Langley (1999) reminds us, the analysis of process data poses many challenges. Such data often include data related to the study of events; data that cross multiple units and levels of analysis; data of variable temporal embeddedness; and data that are eclectic. For all these reasons, developing synthetic theory from case-study-based process data is complex (Fitzgerald et al. 2001).

The data generated by qualitative case studies are themselves relatively loose and difficult to bound. Organizational process research, such as we have undertaken, often seeks to analyse patterns in streams of events. But how is an 'event' defined, bounded and analysed? What are the important events on which the researcher wishes to gather data? As Langley (1999) states: 'The analysis of process data requires a means of conceptualising events and of detecting patterns among them.' So even if the overall methodology used in our different studies is similar (i.e. comparative case studies), the focus of the individual study may determine the particular events to which researchers pay most attention. Thus the nature of the EBHC-based innovations examined varied subtly across the studies.

While all the studies focused on the 'events' generated by the career of evidence-based innovations, three projects (Dopson and Gabbay 1995; Dopson et al. 1999; Locock et al. 1999) concentrated on evidence-based innovations deliberately funded as part of a specific government or regional initiative. The two Warwick studies (Wood et al. 1998; Fitzgerald et al. 1999) focused on evidence-based innovations as they occurred naturally within the normal operation of health care organizations, but sites were selected that were known to have already taken some action on implementing these pieces of evidence. Clinical Standards Advisory Group (CSAG) (CSAG 1998) and Relating Research to Practice (RRTP) (Dawson et al. 1998) also studied naturally occurring innovation. In the two Warwick studies, innovations were selected that were less, as well as more, evidence-based, in order to identify and explain any variation in change outcome.

4.8.2   *Synthesizing data on multiple units and levels of analysis with ambiguous boundaries*

Within case studies of any complexity, data will probably be collected from a number of units, organizational levels, and stakeholders. There are potentially few limits to the data that might be collected. In comparing across cases, we need to be aware of the factors that impinge on the data collection choices made by researchers, particularly where data are thinner or more contained in some cases than others. Funding constraints may well mean that there is pressure on researchers to use less resource-intensive methods. Compare, for example, the reliance on telephone interviews in the evaluations of the PACE project and the Welsh national demonstration projects, with the multiple methods, including on-site 'inspections', of the CSAG project, which inevitably affect the depth and quality of data collection. Such constraints may be imposed on researchers undertaking short-term, policy-relevant research, usually commissioned by institutional funders seeking a clear pragmatic and timely message from the results. This leads to a relatively pragmatic methodology within highly applied projects.

4.8.3   *The influence of the theoretical assumptions of researchers and issues of interpretation*

Critically, all researchers come with implicit (if not explicit) theoretical frameworks (and this would include positivistic, biomedical researchers as well as those, like us, operating from more sociological or political perspectives). We stress this point, given the tendency to see the clinical research paradigm as value-free and objective. In the reflexive world of qualitative and ethnographic research, the subjectivity of researchers needs careful thought and explicit discussion. Our two teams included researchers whose academic backgrounds are in organizational analysis, medical sociology, social policy, and public health. The intellectual similarities within the team were much greater than the differences. None of us would subscribe to a rationalist model of OB and we would generally adopt a political perspective, but would place varying emphasis on the importance, for instance, of notions of culture, power, and structure in explaining what we find. Indeed, we would probably use all of those factors at different times, depending on the context we are researching. However, we have not always been explicit in stating our theoretical perspectives at the outset, either to each other within the team, or when publishing our results. They formed part of a 'taken-for-granted' assumption that we were close enough theoretically to be able to work together.

These (admittedly slight) differences in conceptual and theoretical viewpoints may cause researchers to pay more attention to some types of data than others, even though one attempts to provide cross-checks in the research process. For instance, one might ask individual team members to do independent analysis and then compare the results, both in respect of finding supporting data and especially disconfirming data.

At an interstudy level, there is the question of how far we mean the same thing when we use the same terms in our analysis. When both teams describe scientific evidence as 'socially constructed', do we share the same understanding of what this term means? Even when we attempted to clarify our definitions more explicitly as part of the process of synthesis, we tended to use yet more subjective language to explain the definition and found it difficult to come up with precise definitions. This need to build a common use of concepts across the two teams has also been apparent in our joint work on opinion leaders (Ferlie et al. 2001), where the two teams initially operationalized the concept in slightly different ways.

Our two research teams adopted different terms, with the Warwick team preferring 'champions' or 'product champions', and the Templeton/Southampton team preferring 'opinion leaders'. This gives rise to a number of observations. It implies that we started with somewhat different theoretical perspectives. The term 'product champion' is rooted more firmly in management studies, especially diffusion of innovation studies, whilst the term 'opinion leader' reflects a more mixed approach stemming from both innovation studies and social influence theory. However, these different perspectives were implicit, and we had probably not been aware of this difference between the two teams until we started to examine the topic in detail across the studies.

Both research teams had in practice explored the issue of hostile reactions among key players. However, the Templeton/Southampton team had explicitly encompassed these within their definition of 'opinion leader', whereas the Warwick team had preferred the term 'product champion' and dealt with hostile stakeholders as a separate issue. It required a trawl through each report or article to pick up possibly relevant material.

This perhaps raises a question about how far one can 'systematically' review material when such different terms and definitions are in use, and the reviewer is, in part, acting as a translator. Different subjective understandings of these terms on the part of each research team (let alone each individual researcher) will have affected the way questions about opinion leaders were constructed and asked, and the way in which responses were interpreted and categorized. Furthermore, respondents will also have brought their own subjective understandings to bear. At a broader level, a review of the literature on opinion leaders undertaken by the Templeton/Southampton team has revealed that the problem of inconsistent definitions is widespread and is not confined to health care research (Locock 2001). It is unlikely that the goal of a single replicable description is realistically achievable; the best we can strive for is to make our definitions more explicit both in designing and reporting our research. Of course the task was made easier in the present overview as the teams were able to discuss and explore their differing assumptions—which could only be tentatively inferred if one were simply reviewing the written data. An important implication here is that reports of such studies should aim to be more explicit about their theoretical basis than they usually are at present.

4.9   Concluding remarks

This methodological chapter has considered issues of research paradigm and associated method in HSR, distinguishing between positivistic and interpretive paradigms. We argued that while it is useful to talk of signs of 'rigour' within qualitative research, such indicators are likely to be very different from the hierarchy of evidence model found within the positivistic paradigm. Conversations about what might constitute rigorous qualitative research have begun, but they are still in a relatively early stage.

A frequent objection to qualitative research has been in relation to low levels of external validity. 'Upscaling' qualitative work by taking an overview across a set of similar studies is one response to this criticism so as to produce a more cumulative empirical and theoretical base than is possible within a single case design. This is only methodologically appropriate when all the studies in the set being compared are broadly similar. We outlined a set of seven case-study-based surveys we have undertaken on the careers of EBHC ideas and innovations and argued that they were broadly similar in nature. Nevertheless, we believe this to be a set of cases which, when taken together, are of unusual scope and scale. Another unusual feature has been the opportunity to discuss and debate our material together over an extensive period of time. Subsequent chapters will explore the key themes that emerged from our work together. In these chapters we use abbreviations for the projects rather than full references of the final reports. These are listed in Appendix 4.1.

Appendix 4.1   Project labels

1. Project GR = GRiPP project, Dopson and Gabbay 1995
2. Project Acute = Acute project, Warwick, Wood et al. 1998
3. Project AC/PC = Acute/Primary Care project, Dawson et al. 1998
4. Project CSAG = CSAG project, CSAG 1998
5. Project PC = Primary Care project, Fitzgerald et al. 1999
6. Project PACE = PACE project, Dopson et al. 1999
7. Project WNDP = Wales project, Locock et al. 1999

5

The Active Role of Context

Sue Dopson and Louise Fitzgerald

5.1 Introduction

In Chapter 3, we dwelt on the rise of evidence-based health care (EBHC) policy and practice and discussed responses to the so-called 'implementation gap'—a term referring to the challenges those working within the health care field have in complying with the tenets of evidence-based practice. We questioned the view that the 'gap' could be closed by generic organizational interventions and raised the need for an alternative social perspective, citing emerging work that put forward the uncontroversial point that the social context in which such interventions are targeted invariably plays an important role. Most seasoned commentators on attempts to change practice refer to context as an important influence, but they disagree on the most appropriate way to consider the role of context. Unfortunately, the term 'context' has seldom been explored analytically in health care organizational studies in any depth. It is an important but poorly understood mediator of change and innovation in health care organizations. In this chapter, we will discuss in general terms the ways in which the term 'context' has been formulated and explored within organizational studies as a whole, and also more specifically within the narrower literature on health care organizations. We then present some empirical data, which illuminate aspects of context that we found influential in explaining the career of the EBHC ideas and innovations we studied.

The argument we are seeking to develop in this chapter is that a more sophisticated and active notion of context is needed than is displayed in existing literature if we are to adequately understand the 'implementation gap'. Chapter 8 takes this argument further and seeks, via a number of vignettes from our studies, to give a more detailed flavour of the active role of context in diffusion of innovation.

5.2   Context and organizational studies

Within organizational studies, the term 'context' has been discussed in a number of different ways. Our purpose here is not to simply list the competing theories of how context should be 'properly' formulated, but to reflect on the nature and adequacy of these different formulations. As we discussed in Chapter 2, the overall field of organizational studies comprises a diversity of theoretical preferences and a variety of methods pertaining to appropriate ways of researching social and organizational phenomena. In considering the social phenomena of context, those theorists preferring a more positivist outlook see context as a reality that can be observed and measured easily. At the other extreme there are those in the subjectivist camp, who argue that context is complex and not at all easily assessed and probably not quantifiable at all. Indeed an extreme example of this latter perspective would argue that context is a socially constructed phenomenon and can only be understood by exploring the power relationships that serve to shape what is perceived by organizational actors as relevant contexts.

Contingency theory is an example of a school within organizational studies that explores context in more positivistic terms. This perspective assumes attributes of the environment, including associated technologies, in which organizations sit, and which interact to restrict the range of viable or appropriate organizational forms. Furthermore, it seeks to explain the structure of organizations and individual action by analysing the ways in which organizations adjust to external factors or 'contingencies' that are labelled context. The primary argument of contingency theory is that when an environment is highly stable, a bureaucratic or 'mechanistic' form of organization is functional. The fixed structure of bureaucracy is, however, undermined in more volatile environments when environmental contingencies generate high levels of uncertainty. Organizations in unstable environments, or those using rapidly changing technologies, display patterns of interdependency that are characterized by large numbers of non-routine problems, whose solutions have implications for many parts of the organization (Burns and Stalker 1961) and include the adoption of a more fluid or 'organic' organizational form. Woodward (1965) similarly traced the relationship between particular work technologies and associated organizational forms.

This rather deterministic view of context plays down, for example, the ability of managerial action or perceptions to influence behaviour in organizations and organizational actors' definitions of the context in which they sit. Such a view has also been criticized for operating a reductionist analysis (Meyer et al. 1993: 1177) and has led to a more interpretive view of 'context'. Child and Smiths' work (1987: 590) further exposes the inadequacy of a deterministic view of context. They acknowledge that the appreciation of context is mediated by diverse individual views; this accords organizational actors a degree of strategic choice in the enactment of context. In their case study of Cadbury Limited, three aspects are seen to influence this enactment process: (*a*) objective conditions, for example research and development (R&D) intensity, market concentration; (*b*) the cognitive arena with which its members identify; and (*c*) the network of potential and actual collaborators.

An important perspective in organizational studies that seeks to explore the concept of context with some subtlety is that of organizational configuration (Meyer et al. 1993). The concept of configuration denotes 'any multi-dimensional constellation of conceptually distinct characteristics that commonly occur together' and that 'can be situated at multiple levels of analysis, depicting patterns across individuals, groups, departments and organizations or networks of organizations' (Meyer et al. 1993: 1175). For theorists taking the configurational perspective of context, this potential variety in configuration is limited by the attributes' tendency to fall into coherent patterns.

Academics have suggested that many contextual forces are capable of causing organizational attributes to cluster systematically. For example, there is the perspective of environmental selection within ecological models (Aldrich 1979; Hannan and Freeman 1977, 1989). Here the argument is that while the capacity to take actions consistent with the survival of the organization may rest within the single organization, the rules for selecting 'the survivors' emerge from the sector as a whole, and the sector should be seen as the dominant context.

Institutional theory offers another explanation for uniform configurations. A central argument of this perspective is that the adoption of innovation is not a means of improving performance but is, rather, a means of achieving legitimacy within the organizational field (DiMaggio and Powell 1983: 154). The choice to adopt may, therefore, relate more to institutional pressures associated with certain fads and fashions than to well-founded evidence to support their use. This perspective assumes that conditions of uncertainty in relation to environmental forces, goals, and technical efficiencies will lead organizations to imitate other organizations. Abrahamson (1991) suggests that business schools and consulting firms have a profound influence on the selection of fashionable administrative models.

Another explanation offered for the clustering of organizational attributes lies in the academic tradition of social constructionism. Here the view is that context is the result of the replication of time-honoured practices that become what people know as reality in their everyday lives (Berger and Luckmann 1966). Configuration theory in its many forms pushes us to consider context in a more heuristic fashion. As a general perspective, it has been subject to similar criticisms levelled against contingency theory, namely as offering a reductionist analysis and failing to deal adequately with the role of human action.

Organizational studies also offers a psychological perspective on context. For example, Weick (1969) argues that 'external conditions only become known through the perceptions of organizational members', so that context is fundamentally a mental concept. For Weick (1969: 64), 'the human creates the environment to which the [organizational] system then adapts'. A form of this position is taken by writers such as Smircich and Stubbart (1985) and Meek (1988), who see context as wholly enacted through the social construction of actors. For example, organizational culture as a context for action is viewed as an enacted concept and as a result difficult, if not impossible, to change (Meek 1988: 293).

Context has also been considered within organizational studies in terms of the 'appropriate' levels of analysis that include the environment, the organizational, the individual, and the group. McNulty and Ferlie (2002), reflecting on the analysis of complex new public management (NPM) style reforms to the National Health Service (NHS), recapitulate the levels of the analytical view of context. They posit three broad dimensions of context and argue that all three need to be considered:

1. The macro level of context of the public sector, where three NPM-related contextual forces are stressed as being of particular importance, namely the strength and impact of quasi-market forces, the growth of managerial and clinical managerial roles, and the growth of strategic management.

2. The meso level of context (House et al. 1995), which draws attention to the dynamics of the intermediate level, for example the organizational form of a hospital.
3. The micro level of context, where the emphasis is on the history and dynamics of activity within particular clinical settings in the hospital.

McNulty and Ferlie use these three levels of context to explore the career and impact of a Business Process Re-engineering Change Programme in an NHS trust hospital and 'trace the downward links between them'. An example of the way in which the perception of macro context shaped hospitalwide action was in the managerial assessment that the introduction of the internal market as a new national policy would create local conditions of severe competition, in which traditional incremental savings would be insufficient and in which radical approaches to redesign would be needed (in fact, this assessment of the macro context proved in the end to be over-pessimistic). Empirically, this study revealed the way in which the perception of wider context influenced the corporate response, which then influenced the response of the intermediate tier (clinical directorate) and then the clinical setting. It did not, however, explore ways in which the people acted—or might have acted—to reshape the wider environmental context.

From this purposefully general review of the ways in which context has been considered in organizational studies, it is clear that there are different approaches from which to choose. There is, however, a danger of becoming trapped in unproductive arguments as to whether context is best considered as an objective entity or can only be understood in a more subjectivist fashion. We should not be surprised that the debates on context exist in such a form within organizational studies; after all, for years sociologists have been debating whether society or the individual is more real and which should come first as a point of departure in sociological investigation. Such polarity of debate is also found within discussions of research methodology, as discussed in Chapter 4. Research is often described in such all-or-nothing terms, which means either totally 'objective' or, conversely, completely lacking objectivity, that is, as being subjective in an absolute sense.

There have been a number of important theoretical contributions that question the historical dualism of structure and agency. For example, Child's work (1972, 1997) on strategic choice combines an awareness of objective environment and the possibility of management action as well as Giddens' formulation of structuration theory (Giddens 1984). Structuration is a term that refers to the dynamic articulation between structure and action (which Giddens called 'agency'). Giddens argues that organizational theories have treated structure as an exogenous constraint on action, and have viewed action as independent of structure. In organizational studies, the implicit gulf between structure and action is reflected in the distinction between micro- and macro-organizational behaviour (OB). Giddens argues that action and structure are inextricably linked, that action both 'constitutes and is constituted by' structure. Actions may therefore replicate, but may also alter existing structural patterns. Structuration is important in organizational studies because it provides a theoretical and empirical base for bridging the gulf between studies of organizational structure and studies of everyday action in organizations.

Drawing on structuration theory, the Centre for Corporate Strategy and Change, led by Pettigrew (1985, 1987) in the late 1980s and early 1990s, provided an important contribution to the field of organizational analysis and the discussion of context, by virtue of the considerable body of research and writing generated on strategic change processes. Pettigrew (1985) encouraged his researchers to undertake research 'which is contextual and processual in character'. In Pettigrew's terms, a contextualist analysis of a social process 'draws on phenomena at vertical and horizontal levels of analysis and the interconnections between those levels through time'. Here, the vertical level refers to the interdependencies between higher or lower levels of analysis upon phenomena, for example the impact of a changing socio-economic context on features of intraorganizational context and interest-group behaviour. The horizontal level refers to the sequential interconnectedness among phenomena in historical, present, and future time. More specifically he argues that a wholly 'contextualist' analysis would exhibit the following characteristics:

1. A clearly delineated but theoretically and empirically connectable set of levels of analysis.
2. A clear description of the processes under investigation at a system and action level.
3. A theory that specifies a view on human behaviour.
4. A linkage of the contextual variables in the vertical analysis to the processes under observation in the horizontal analysis.

Pettigrew's starting point for the analysis of change is that any new initiative inevitably involves managing both an outer and inner context and process. Outer context refers to the social, economic, political, and competitive environment in which the organization operates. Inner context refers to the structure, corporate culture, history, and political environment in the organization, within which ideas for change have to proceed.

This general approach has also been associated with the tradition of process research, itself described as the dynamic study of behaviour within organizations, focusing on the core themes of organizational context, activities, and actions that unfold over time (Pettigrew 1990). The handling of time distinguishes process research from other methods, which are more cross-sectional in nature. Process research seeks to identify trends or patterns of association rather than predictive laws (Pawson and Tilley 1997), and stipulates that because processes are embedded in outer or inner contexts, the interaction between context and human action should be the focus of study. Pettigrew et al. (1992) point out that the existing NHS literature base is weakened because it is insufficiently processual (an emphasis on action as well as structure); comparative; pluralist (a description and analysis of the often competing versions of reality seen by actors in change processes); contextual (operating at a variety of different levels with specification of the linkages between them); and historical (taking into account the historical evolution of ideas and stimuli for change as well as the constraints within which decision-makers operate).

Langley's overview (1999) of process methods in organizational studies reveals the radically different approaches that can be undertaken. This would include not only traditional forms of narrative-based process research reviewed here but also more quantitative forms (Scott Poole et al. 2000) of analysis. However, this latter approach appears to lose the strong internal validity and holistic portrayal of a phenomenon, which might be thought to be the distinctive strength of process research. McNulty and Ferlie's work (2002) constitutes a text that exemplifies the recent application of process research methods to the study of a complex NHS change programme over time.

These more analytical discussions of health care context are a welcome relief from discussions that see context as a layered and unidirectional set of influences (see Figure 5.1) where the outer layer involves influences from government health policy, which moves

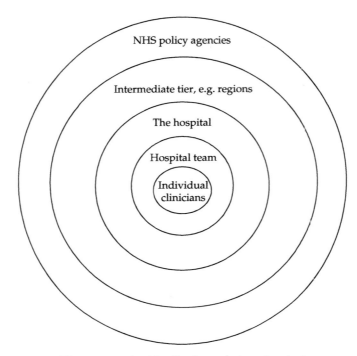

Figure 5.1 *A misleading layered view of context*

down to regional/local influences and finally to influences specific to a single organization and individual practitioners.

As already suggested, there are three difficulties of such a unidirectional view of context. Firstly, organizations, groups, and individuals are portrayed as passive recipients subject to aspects of health care context that shape behaviour, but with no leeway in choosing which aspects of context to bring into the organization and with no influence with which they could reshape the context. Secondly, these contexts are somehow separated out rather than treated as an 'integrated configuration'. Thirdly, such a view implies a static view of context, that is, context is seen as a particular setting at a particular point in time rather than as evolving and changing over time.

We are not alone in recognizing these difficulties; Fitzgerald et al. (2002) seek to reconceptualize the bringing in of context into organizational action using health care data. Their data draw attention to the interplay of features of the outer and inner context and note multiple differences of value, structures, education, and relationships between the acute and primary sectors of health care. They conclude:

Ultimately, the behaviour of the stakeholders and the features of context are interlocked. The combination of multilayered, two-way influences, multiple stakeholders with interpretative schemes, innovation-seeking behaviour by individuals and groups, and differing absorptive capacity in organizations produces a situation in which context is an actor. (Fitzgerald et al. 2002)

5.3 Aspects of context that influence the career of EBHC initiatives

Some interesting patterns emerge from the review of our data on this issue. A first observation is the relatively low profile of managerial stakeholders in the diffusion processes studied. Indeed in Project PACE and Project WNDP, this was true despite the projects being sponsored by them. Given the operation of quasi-market forces at the time the data were gathered, we expected that the contracting process would constitute an important aspect of context. However, there is little evidence across the studies that this proved significant. Users or patients were rarely mentioned as a major influence on the career of an initiative.

At the meso level of context, we would expect the intermediate bodies operating between government policy and practitioners to play an important part in the diffusion processes studied across the projects. The regional role (now replaced by the strategic health authority [SHA]) has changed radically over the last five years. In essence, the region's role has moved away from being a tiered direct-line management body to one offering specialist functions in research and development, medical education, as well as the board of strategic oversight of health care. Yet the 'regional office' was rarely mentioned as an important aspect of context in our data. The general impression was that the region was distant and remote from clinical work. That said, the main regionally organized network, post-graduate continuing education, was seen as impacting on the diffusion process. For example, in Project PC, many general practitioners (GPs) used this network as the way in which they kept up to date with new research.

I think they (postgraduate meetings) are starting to become good. Postgraduate education is probably one of those areas where there is a fair amount of cross-boundary contact between professionals—I think it works particularly well in area 'x' because we have a number of our GPs who are in the educational field. (Project PC, HAPC leader)

HAs, in their position between government policy-makers and prac-titioners, are in theory well placed to play a more active role in innovation and diffusion processes. The actual role HAs played across the studies was perceived by respondents as limited, again despite the fact that in Project PACE and Project WNDP HAs were, in effect, sponsors of the projects.

Whilst the HA was rarely referred to as being a key influence in the diffusion of innovations across the projects, the public health depart-ment was often mentioned as an important source of information about research. For example, the production of a digest of evidence-based medicine (EBM) from public health was welcomed by the GPs in the primary care study (Project PC) and was deemed an important tool for them to keep in touch with recent research, and therefore an influence on practice. Interviewees in Project GR readily acknow-ledged the role of public health in the four projects. Indeed as one of the first pilot projects exploring the ways in which the results of research might influence practice in the country, Project GR was effectively championed by public health physicians with two of the projects being led by them.

Stronger contextual influences discussed in the data included ac-cess to groups and networks and, in particular, professional net-works. For example, across Project AC/PC, Project Acute, and Project PC, the Royal Colleges and professional bodies emerge as important sources of information with respect to research evidence, but not as particularly influential in directly facilitating changes in practice. Likewise, specialist bodies such as Aggressive Research Intelligence Facility (ARIF), the Cochrane Centre, and the Centre for the dissemination of EBM were often referred to as providing add-itional helpful sources of information. The Royal Colleges, profes-sional associations, and specialist information organizations remain important in developing and shaping the nature of clinical education as seen by professionals and, therefore, as part of the wider context, they did play a role in shaping clinical behaviour and thus influencing the career of the initiative. Professions and professional work are, of course, a key feature of health care contexts and are discussed fully in Chapter 6.

In Project Acute, the marketing function of drug and equipment firms often proved to be an influence on the career of the innovation studied. For example, the new generation of low-molecular-weight heparins (LMWHs) was under patent and marketed by the drug companies.

It was only as a result of drug company publicity that we ever heard of LMWHs. There was a great deal of drug company money thrown about at that time. There were free lunches. The whole drug company marketing effort went in to getting us to use these rather expensive chemicals on a regular or universal basis. (Project Acute, consultant surgeon)

New networks formed due to national policy shifts also proved to impact on the career of some of the innovations studied. For example, the out-of-hours cooperative networks of GPs formed to deal with emergencies across a geographical area 'out of hours', which resulted in new groupings and informal exchange of information amongst the primary care commissioners.

Fundholding has made a difference because we are members of a multi-fund. And that has pulled in 8 or 10 practices, maybe more. The most disparate, odd set of GPs who you would not imagine would mix, and yet we have been a superb group because we had that common aim. (Project PC, GP)

A key mediating factor in securing changes in clinical practice appeared as the extent to which clinicians had access to membership of groups. Not only are groups the arena for sharing experience and facilitating learning, they are also an important means through which formal communication from literature, guidelines, and educational initiatives is filtered. There were several examples of group arrangements that proved helpful in facilitating change. Commissioning groups, comprising representatives of GPs from both fund-holding and non-fund-holding practices played a critical role in drawing GPs into strategic decision-making and setting districtwide priorities for care. Postgraduate meetings proved to be useful as interactive places for validating information, although often respondents would make the point that unless the practitioner who is presenting the information is someone who could be respected by the participant, it was likely to be disregarded. Education networks acted as a forum for exchange of information that sometimes facilitated the diffusion process. For example:

The best forum for me in meeting other GP innovators over the last ten to fifteen years has been as a college examiner, where two or three times a year you meet with a group of examiners from all over the country to run the exam. There is no better forum really to know what is going on in other places. Most of the people who are interested in that kind of activity are fairly energetic. (Project PC, GP)

Audit machinery was another example of a useful forum for group discussion and decision that impacted on changing clinical practice:

At an audit meeting a long time ago, it was felt that we should do something and we discussed what we should do, and we came to the decision that we should do Heparin? (Project Acute, consultant orthopaedic surgeon)

It was a drag at the time (audit), but we went in ourselves to audit and understood there were practical problems.... More debate is generated by focus on current practice locally, rather than uncontroversial hard truth or evidence. (Project PACE, project leader)

An important meso level influence appeared unsurprisingly as the structure and organization of the acute and primary care (AC/PC) sector. Essentially hospitals operate in a hierarchical fashion. Care is organized in relation to specialities run by clear hierarchies within particular groups. Primary care has a number of distinctive contextual features. In particular, there is a vast complexity of reporting relationships, accountabilities, interprofessional boundaries, and interorganizational linkages. It is more aptly described as a network of organizations. Its specific features include fragmentation, loosely coupled small units, and GP practices that are essentially partnerships. These units have links to a wider array of other organizations, to each other, to the HA, to the acute centre, to the community trust, and to social services.

Professional relationships and boundaries significantly mediate structural and organizational arrangements in health care. For example, the hierarchical structures in hospitals meant that junior doctors in Project AC/PC felt constrained to use the evidence their seniors told them to. The junior doctors' knowledge base for the clinical routines on the wards or outpatients was, therefore, always subordinated to the views of their seniors. Such power relationships were among the most obvious mediators of whether a given piece of evidence was 'sticky' or flowed freely down particular organizational channels. (In this case there was pressurized flow down the channels, with authority, respect, and deference acting—to pursue the metaphor—as valves that prevented retrograde flow up the vertical hierarchical channels.) Such channels of authority and hierarchy were also an important way in which local internal opinion leaders had influence. Where the 'boss' of a firm had formed a strong opinion that a certain new practice was appropriate, he or she had, as part of the medical profession's ethos and working practices, well-established hierarchical channels through which to ensure that all the clinicians in 'his' (or 'her') team understood the requirement to comply even where they may disagree. The consultants' knowledge would therefore flow easily down such channels even where there might be some intellectual resistance such as a concern that those views might be idiosyncratic or outdated.

The views of junior doctors about the evidence were not visible in our case studies as sources of change in hospital routines. Yet there is no rational reason why that should have been so. Most junior doctors were either engaged in, or had recently been involved in, professional examinations (membership or fellowship of Royal Colleges), which might be expected to expose them to up to date evidence and leading views on best practice. They would therefore be, if anything, *more* familiar, on average, with cutting-edge explicit codified research evidence than their consultant bosses, albeit they would have relatively much weaker experiential and tacit knowledge. Yet their knowledge of such evidence played almost no part. It was as if the logic of the hierarchy and of superior experience supplanted the logic of up to date research knowledge.

What then if those lower down the hierarchy disagreed with the consultants' view of the explicit evidence, or believed that they had come across contradictory evidence to an extent that they believed the consultant was wrong? How might that influence the eventual implementation of the evidence? We did not directly hear about such instances but must assume from other experience and observations of hospital life that the fate of that contradictory evidence in that particular organization would depend on aspects of the local context, such as how hierarchical that particular clinical firm was, what the impact might be on day-to-day professional activity, how highly regarded the consultant was, what the likely cost consequences might be, whether others within or without the organization were also pressing for the change suggested by the junior doctor and, if so, how strong the consultant's power base was in relation to those pressing for the change. The fate of the new evidence, therefore, would rely on the immediate context within which it was being negotiated—not upon the strength or logic of the junior doctor's evidential base.

Similarly, what if the nursing staff disagreed? The normal hospital hierarchy might make their views subordinate to those of the medical staff, and nurses' views on the evidence base for practices suggested by their doctor colleagues might, therefore, have relatively little impact on its eventual implementation. But sometimes, where senior members of the nursing or midwifery profession disagreed with senior doctors, more subtle methods of persuasion and management could have an impact on practice. These tactics could include the co-opting of allied forces to outweigh the existing power of the key decision-maker.

Or the tactic might be to use managerial pathways to try and persuade colleagues to consider a new set of guidelines from a college, the region, or a national source, in the hope that the ensuing debates and discussion might help overcome the barriers. Attempts to alter practice might also involve bringing influential allies to bear from within the consultant's own respected peer group to try to alter their view. There will be few who work in the hospital sector who will not have experience of the subtle methods by which nursing and allied professions influence the behaviour of doctors—sometimes by virtue of the respect they have earned as team members, but sometimes extending to subterfuge and the equivalent of guerrilla tactics to undermine the boss's authority and powerbase. Part of that struggle for acceptance of their views might rely on demonstrating a greater proficiency as a result of their tacit knowledge about best practice. The respect, for example, that midwives engendered among junior doctors made it more likely that the young doctors would accept their views on debatable topics.

Sapiential authority was thus one means by which entrenched power bases could be overcome in order to facilitate the flow of evidence. No overt challenge on the evidence base of the consultant could succeed unless it came from a source with sufficient authority to command the necessary respect in the eyes of the decision-makers. Non-medical professions had, therefore, to gain the respect of clinical decision-makers if they were to influence their decisions. A clear example was in Project GR, where one public health department expended large resources on a relatively junior researcher to review evidence about stroke care, and recognized in retrospect that the main benefit had not been in the evidence itself (which usually proved in any case to be insufficient to support most of the necessary practical decisions), but rather in the respect that the exercise earned for the public health department and for the principles of systematic reviewing. By this means, the non-clinicians from the public health department were accorded a very persuasive voice, which they believed they would never otherwise have had, in the detailed debates in the design of the local stroke service.

There was an amazing change in our small working group. We got into a clinician-to-clinician barney, and someone suddenly turned and asked [the researcher from public health] 'what's the evidence?' She sat there eventually like the Emperor giving thumbs up and thumbs down! She became the oracle despite being foreign, an AHP [allied health professional], and a woman! (Project GR, public health consultant)

Moreover, the public health team could use this newly earned respect for their knowledge base alongside their well-established managerial links and organizational skills, so that it became an essential part of the range of techniques that enabled them to bring about the changes they desired. We see here a very clear example of how the context of professional hierarchies and boundaries was intimately bound up with the way in which evidence was ascertained, transformed, and used within an organization. Without the respect—and sapiential authority—earned by the public health researcher and capitalized on by the organizational savvy of the public health director, the evidence would never have entered the debates with powerful clinicians, nor resulted in the collectively negotiated changes in the evidence base of their clinical practice.

While hospital organizations had well-established hierarchies, professional networks, and communities of practice that both facilitated and impeded the flow of knowledge, the structures in general practice were quite different. GPs in our case studies had their natural networks of colleagues within their own practices (few in our case studies were single-handed) but also had contact through other groupings, which similarly allowed knowledge to be negotiated and developed iteratively through discussion. Earlier in this chapter, we were told about the usefulness of commissioning groups and fund-holders groups and occasionally audit groups—where clinical pathways were discussed or where priorities for improvement were agreed—in which exchange of views with respected colleagues initiated, accelerated, or stifled the progress of a new idea for improved services. Where GPs were closely involved with such groups and had well-developed networks, and where they also had influence within their own group practice, they were more likely to implement a change grounded on explicit, research-based knowledge or to develop good reasons for rejecting it. As discussed earlier, also important were networks explicitly put in place for education and continuing professional development, where the informal links with colleagues were established and consolidated, allowing ideas to be shared and critically discussed in a relatively casual way. Wider networks (e.g. Royal College of General Practitioners [RCGP] meetings and committees) were also important channels for the flow of knowledge among GP colleagues.

Such meetings were also a way of keeping in touch with the views of the opinion leaders outside the GPs' own immediate circle. Here, as in the hospital, successful management of change required considerable effort by the change team to ensure that GPs came into contact with opinion leaders who favoured the desired change and could argue the case cogently and authoritatively. Where that failed to happen, the results could be counterproductive—as in the instances where GPs found that the consultant opinion leaders either failed to practise what they preached or displayed a lack of understanding of the relevance of their specialist-derived proposals to general practice—when the hospital-based 'expert opinion leaders' rapidly lost ground to the 'peer opinion leaders' among GPs. Again this illustrates how closely the local context (in this case the exposure to genuinely influential opinion leaders) could make all the difference to the uptake of codified research knowledge.

Opinion leaders emerged across the studies as a particularly important aspect of the micro context influencing the career of many of the innovations we studied. In our projects we adopted different terms—champion, project champion, opinion leader—to describe these people. Here the latter term is used to encompass their potential to oppose as well as support a change initiative.

Project Acute concludes:

Professional groupings retained a key role in decision making. Proposals for change driven from outside did not influence local clinical groups where much discretion resided. The learning and change capability of these groups was shaped by prior history and their pattern of roles and relationships. The case for change was enhanced by the presence of clinical 'product champions'.... Such advocates bring credibility and establish leadership within their own professional groupings.

Evidence from Project PC further reinforces the influence of credible change champions. Project AC/PC argues that the influence of colleagues and seniors is one of the 'multiple cues' identified by clinicians as significant in influencing practice. These influences are in a sense absorbed into their own accumulated clinical experience:

[D]octors' own views of their clinical world ... are shaped by a strong sense of their own autonomy to develop practice in accordance with their experience, in which they include encounters with literature, research, opinion formers and seniors, but none of these is seen as dominant over—or in a sense separate from—their experience.

The ability to respond selectively to peer influence is seen as a marker of their professional independence.

The definition and selection of opinion leaders is important, and may be oversimplified; the conclusion in some studies that they have no effect may be undermined if they have not been appropriately defined. Subjective understandings of what an opinion leader is or does can differ substantially in each local setting. All studies found a spread of very different types and categories of opinion leaders: some who were experts and some who were peers; some who were hostile, some who were very positive, and some whose enthusiasm occasionally went too far; some with an ambivalent or hidden agenda; and some who were cynical about what they were doing but did it successfully nonetheless.

Opinion leaders with their own agenda can be damaging. They come forward for a reason—it may be partly out of the goodness of their hearts or an evangelical mission, but they all have vested interests, which may work for you or they may work against you. (Project PACE, project leader)

The evidence from our studies suggests that opinion leaders sit at different points along a number of axes, including, not least, the following:

Technical expert (academic, clinician) ↔ Peer
Formal leadership ↔ Informal/emergent leadership
Supportive ↔ Hostile
Committed ↔ Ambivalent/non-committed
Corporate ↔ Individualist/maverick
Enthusiastic ↔ Disaffected
Optimistic ↔ Cynical
Leading by instruction ↔ Leading by example (e.g. following guidelines)
Conformist ↔ Deviant
Professional/technical ↔ Executive/managerial.

Perceived inconsistencies between what the opinion leader says and what he or she does may have a profound effect on their influence—for example, in projects where opinion leaders in secondary care did not follow the same guidelines they were recommending to GPs, signalling that they preferred to rely on their own clinical judgement as a higher form of knowledge. This illustrates the problem of getting a single replicable description to be used in testing opinion leaders as an intervention to achieve change. It also underlines the importance of being alert to the fact that the opinion leader whose impact is being tested may not be the only local influence on the practitioners concerned, and that the influence of negative or hostile opinion leaders not formally part of a trial may be cancelling out any effect.

Project Acute notes that 'innovations which involved antagonistic or multiple stakeholders...faced difficulties'. Similarly Project WNDP concludes that 'where projects encountered active hostility, some serious problems occurred', including one project where GP leaders almost completely withdrew cooperation from a project that had been progressing well and caused substantial delays in implementation. Project Acute cautions against 'the unwritten assumption that innovation is a positive thing': opinion leaders' opposition to an innovation may in fact be beneficial resistance to an organizationally inappropriate change.

The presence of hostile opinion leaders is one example of a wider problem of isolating other local contextual influences on the change process. Project WNDP suggests:

[A]lthough the support of opinion leaders is helpful, desirable, and even necessary, it is not itself a sufficient condition for change. It is one piece of a locally unique jigsaw, where evidence, peer comparison, clinical experience, interpersonal relationships, concerns about the quality of care, managerial action and funding—to name but a few—also need to fit together.

An opinion leader who works well with one practitioner may fail to make progress with another. Project Acute noted:

[W]here good interpersonal relationships exist there is greater opportunity for modalities of practice to be discussed and a common way forward found. Where this was the Project, our evidence suggests practitioners would be better able to respond to information and decide to change practice or not on the basis of it. Surgeons were far more likely to listen to the views of others whom they thought were important and who in turn thought their point of view was important.

Project WNDP explores the potential to distinguish between two main categories of supportive opinion leaders, which could be described as experts and peers. Inevitably these categories oversimplify, as it is possible to be both a peer and an expert, but one role may be more evident than the other in particular situations.

The expert opinion leader was seen as a higher authority (often an academic or consultant) able to explain the evidence and respond convincingly to challenges and debate, or alternatively whose support for the initiative is itself sufficient endorsement. Their role appeared particularly important in the initial stages of sowing an idea, endorsing the evidence, and translating it into a form which is acceptable to practitioners and takes account of their local experience. However, they might be less suited to following through to implementation and may even provoke some hostility. All studies have noted particular ambivalence towards academic experts, who may be felt to be too remote from the concerns of practitioners to persuade them effectively. Project Acute suggests:

[T]he development of hybrid researcher-practitioner roles (rather than reliance on external scientists) may help. The construction of alliances between researchers and clinicians, where there is feedback in exchange for the enlisting of patients in trials, may also build up 'ownership' of research findings.

The peer opinion leader, particularly in primary care, is seen as someone who has applied the innovation within his or her own practice and can give colleagues confidence that they could do it too. They thus have a stronger role in the later stages of practical implementation.

It makes people think 'the ordinary GP can do it. If he can do it perhaps I can'. It's not just the super-efficient, well-known people. (Project PACE)

There is evidence from several of the studies that new peer opinion leaders, who would not previously have been recognized by their colleagues as educationally influential, could be created or identified, provided they were genuinely credible to their colleagues. The danger of innovators who step too far beyond the current norm to retain their credibility was, however, a recurring theme. Project PC suggests that, especially in primary care, 'to retain their credibility, individual professionals need to continue to practice. One could therefore envisage the development of part-time roles within local contexts'.

Our work suggests that opinion leadership, exercised within that local set of circumstances, is an important influence on the career of EBHC initiatives. As well as the structural or other contextual factors that moderate the relationship, the skills and style of different opinion leaders may affect their ability to persuade others, and the dynamic exchange between two individuals (or more) is vital. Such individuals can use aspects of the context in which they find themselves to influence innovation processes. An illustration of the way opinion leaders used aspects of context to achieve change is from Project PC, where GPs used their budgets to employ physiotherapists despite the lack of evidence. Other pieces of evidence, such as clinical experience and patient feedback, were used to defend the introduction of the innovation.

We found many examples in our data where practitioners reinterpreted the financial or physical environment in which they practise, which will then constitute another aspect of the context and shape how they change their policy. For example, in Project PC, the decision as to whether the GPs could afford a community physiotherapist was a judgement that then became a contextual reason for adopting such a service. In the event, they decided that they would accept very weak research evidence in favour of using a community physiotherapy service because it was their collective perception of the context that the demand from their patients and the affordability of the service made for a favourable context. But they need not necessarily have enacted such a favourable context, and indeed other stakeholders, for example the HA, did not agree with that perception, and saw the context differently. Had the GPs decided, like the HA, that the opportunity costs of the physiotherapists were too high and the resources would be more effective elsewhere, or noted that many patients actually preferred, say, chiropraxy, then they may have seen the same level of weak research evidence as a reason for rejecting the new service.

5.4   What are the building blocks of a more sophisticated notion of context?

Thus far we have simply considered aspects of 'context' our research participants reported as influential on the career of the innovations we studied. There are, of course, dangers in relying on such data. The importance of a more detailed analysis is well illustrated in Project AC/PC. Here the 256 clinicians interviewed were quite dismissive of the place of organizational and managerial considerations in influencing their clinical practice. Yet within this study a number of inherited organizational arrangements such as the nature of the screening arrangements; the involvement of clinicians in groups where practice and evidence are discussed; the fact that medical careers are developed within relatively strict hierarchical structures, which means that juniors have to practice within the guidelines of seniors whether they agree with these guidelines or not; the composition of particular services; the extent to which community services are integrated with hospital services; the nature of the referral and knowledge of its significance; and knowledge of waiting lists, all appear important, if unacknowledged, influences on individual practice and the career of innovation.

Another general feature of interviewees' responses across all the studies was the extent to which they were often unaware of how past events impacted on the present context of which they were a part. Interesting initial material illustrating this point is from Project AC/ PC. One case in this project explored the treatment of glue ear in children. The services studied had been formed over a long period of time, rather than being a recent invention. For example, the large audiology service in one site (code-named Wisteria) emerged as a result of the efforts of a charismatic audiologist in the 1970s. In another site (Holly) the children's hearing clinic was located in the Ear, Nose, and Throat (ENT) because the clinician in charge developed the service there some years ago. A separate ENT audiology service existed on the same site, but there was little exchange of information between them. It is within a particular inherited organizational context, such as the two examples given here, that the groups involved have negotiated patterns of practice that become shared and understood as the way a condition is treated. This understanding is often re-negotiated as one group or an individual seeks to make change. The inherited organizational arrangements, coupled with the complex interdependencies between groups, constituted significant disincentives to more strategic change.

In our view there are a number of building blocks that help us in the quest for a more sophisticated and active notion of context. A more sophisticated notion must acknowledge that local contexts are multidimensional, multifaced configurations of forces. For example, the hospital trust is crucially influenced by the arrangements for primary care and social services. Furthermore, no 'context' is discrete. There are complex connections and interactions that individuals often are not aware of. The diagrammatic representation of the referral paths and potential waiting points for glue ear (Figure 5.2) demonstrates the complexity of the relevant local contexts involved in the treatment of glue ear.

In addition, managerial groups might also affect treatment patterns. For example, purchasers in the glue ear case in Project AC/PC were in a position to refuse to finance grommet insertion (this happened in one HA in the study) or to impose conditions, which must be adhered to before such operations could be carried out. Purchasers were also able to affect organizational arrangements, for example by agreeing to finance larger or smaller community audiology departments. Public health physicians influenced glue ear management as they formulated screening policies for the HA. Trust management could influence particular staffing issues within the hospital, operating of course within the wider policy and resource context.

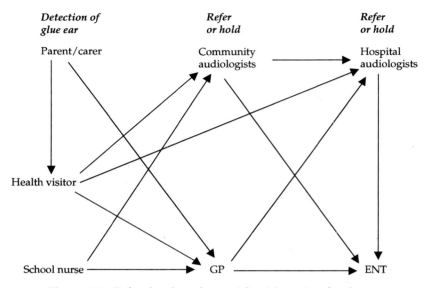

Figure 5.2   *Referral paths and potential waiting points for glue ear*

This extended example of glue ear shows how organizational actors in the NHS are not isolated individuals. Individuals live within, and are a part of, a network of social relationships that extend well beyond the organization to which they, in name, belong. Furthermore such actors have been, and continue to be, influenced by the shadow of past periods and historic decisions, which they have inherited. This aspect of the creation and development of context has been under-researched, but in our data has been demonstrated to be critical, and crucially needs to inform a more sophisticated notion of context. History may help explain the differentiation and the variations between health care units of an organization that are nominally performing the same tasks in the same circumstances. A more sophisticated notion of context must also acknowledge the capacity of individuals to influence context. Actors perceive and interpret aspects of context in different ways. In practice, individuals do not view the facets of context as separate; rather they experience them as a maelstrom, or at least a morass. Individuals seek to make sense of multiple contexts drawing on a mixture of cognitive and emotional judgement to create an 'integral context', and it is with this in mind that action takes place. Yet the ways in which actors construe their environment is a social act. Collectively, they make sense of their context and thereby create, or 'enact' (Weick 1995), that environment, which in turn impacts upon the actors' ability or willingness to effect the change.

Many clinicians in our case studies felt bombarded by guidelines received from the centre of the NHS or their professional bodies, by managerial imperatives from their own employers, or by new research published in the journals—not to mention all the interesting developments they might pick up at conferences and meetings. They did not simply respond passively to this multitude of ideas. Rather they actively selected and modified them in the light of their perceived demands, constraints, and freedom to act. Context looked different from the perspective of the various clinicians and managers who were involved in the change process, because each from their own perspective was selecting and prioritizing their environment in differing ways. For example, from the management point of view, NHS performance targets might loom large, whereas for the clinicians they might safely be ignored compared to the demands of their professional ethos. As an organization, the key actors needed to make sense of their environment collectively and, therefore, even the environment within which they operated—the demands from the Department of Health (DoH), the local financial constraints, the acceptability of current levels of performance, the relevance of a new research finding in the *British Medical Journal*, the relative influence of the clinical director and the director of public health—creates a form of negotiated reality.

To decide which evidence-based practices should be adopted was, therefore, anything but a simple matter of seeking out the appropriate evidence and persuading colleagues to use it. There was an element both of 'push' and 'pull' (Williams and Gibson 1990) in these processes. Usually someone—not necessarily one of the clinicians—had formed the view that there was good available evidence that was not being implemented. But many of our interviewees also commented that it was important to have a feeling among the practitioners in the organization that the evidence related to an area of practice where they saw a need for improvement in the quality of care. This perception could come from many quarters, but ultimately it needed to be accepted by the clinicians if the 'pull' element was to play a part.

[M]ost people are only basically concerned with their own patch... if we'd gone to [hospital X] or something and said look this is anticoagulation and these are the issues, they would have been asleep in five minutes because it's not a hot issue; they are not interested; why bother? (Project Acute, consultant)

More importantly, there were some instances in which the perception of the need for change lowered the threshold for what was considered appropriate evidence.

There wasn't strong evidence but it didn't matter—the perception of need was important. (Project PACE, health promotion adviser)

There's not much evidence in this area at all actually. The reasons to go in for this kind of work [i.e. the intended change in practice] are humanitarian. (Project PACE, consultant physician)

In these and similar cases where there was a desire to improve the quality of a service, individuals used the general promotion of evidence-based practice as an opportunistic way of capturing the interest of the colleagues. For example, in one of the PACE projects, there had been little local interest or sense of urgency in improving a Cinderella service, where standards were poor. The purpose of bidding for PACE funds was deliberately to create a perception among the clinicians that there was an 'evidence-based' need for a change in the way patients were managed and to use the PACE initiative and funding to secure that improvement. Yet there was actually not a great deal of relevant research evidence to underpin the desired improvement.

5.5   Concluding remarks

Our empirical findings lend considerably more weight to claims concerning the importance of 'context' on the career of innovations. The data also confirm the view put forward by Fitzgerald et al. (2002) and others that context needs to be better integrated into the analysis of diffusion processes. Specifically our data retest these ideas on a much larger, more diverse, population of organizations and produce more generalizable findings because of the reflection process we went through, as described in Chapter 4. Configuration and structuration theories highlight the interplay between structure and process; they perhaps do not acknowledge the role of human action as fully as is needed. We have suggested in this chapter that context should not be seen as a backcloth to action but as an interacting element in the diffusion process.

We have argued that more sophisticated models of context must acknowledge that local contexts are multifaceted, multidimensional configurations of forces which often interact in complex ways that invariably lead to unintended consequences. Furthermore, a model of context must acknowledge that context is socially perceived and enacted and is, therefore, actively brought into processes of innovation. Health professionals do not simply apply abstract, disembodied scientific research rigidly to the situation around them. Instead they collaborate in discussion, relate the evidence to the context, and engage in work practices that actively interpret and (re)construct its local validity and usefulness. That activity is rarely carried out by individuals in isolation and often includes the redefinition of the context within which the practitioners will assess the evidence.

In the next chapter we look in more depth at a key aspect of health care contexts, the critical role played by professions and professionals in interpreting and translating evidence into practice.

6

Professional Boundaries and the Diffusion of Innovation

Louise Fitzgerald and Sue Dopson

6.1 Introduction

In Chapter 5, we illustrated the crucial interrelationship between the context and the career of the diffusion of an innovation. In this chapter, we extend our analysis to examine the impact of professional boundaries as an important aspect of context on the career of evidence-based health care (EBHC) initiatives. The multiprofessional nature of health care has been identified as an important characteristic that has implications for the implementation of policy, for top-down change, and for the improvement of quality standards and care and also for the movement of knowledge across different occupational groupings.

To focus on the effect of professional boundaries on the diffusion process in health care settings, we shall first review selected aspects of the wider literature on the professions. We begin with a brief history of the way in which the study of the system of professions has developed in the literature. This underlines that this system of relationships is framed by time and changing social, structural relations. The remainder of the discussion focuses on four key topics: power, professional jurisdiction, and the State; the role of knowledge in securing and maintaining professional status; the part played by professional socialization in diffusion; and the impact of the boundaries between professionals and managers.

As Dopson (1993) and Blackler et al. (1993) argue, there is a need to consolidate the differing perspectives on professions, drawn from the historical and sociological traditions. One immediate outcome of a retrospective review is that it highlights the fact that the focus of research has been predominantly on the medical profession. So far, there have been limited attempts to compare professions or to examine other clinical professions beyond medicine (Etzioni 1969; Larkin 1979). Nonetheless, many authors have offered historical over-views of developments in the literature of the professions (Becker 1962; Parkin 1979; Saks 1983; Blackler et al. 1993; Exworthy and Half-ord 1999). These reviews demonstrate the shift in thinking from early work that tended to focus on defining the characteristics of profes-sions and their unique or 'special' qualities to more critical perspec-tives. The early work might be defined as the trait or taxonomic school, after Klegon (1978). However, as Saks points out, it was increasingly clear that this perspective was obscuring the social and historical conditions under which occupational groups became pro-fessions—including the power struggles involved in the process of professionalization. The trait school can, therefore, be seen as essen-tially ahistorical and acontextual, uncritically promoting the attri-butes of professional organization used to ensure tight boundaries around work.

Critical and alternative approaches came from the neo-Weberian school, so called because these writers sought to apply the Weberian concept of social closure to professional occupations. Of importance here is the focus on the power dimension, since this aligns with our interest in interprofessional or occupational boundaries. Writers in this school (Berlant 1975; Parry and Parry 1976; Parkin 1979) identify two forms of closure: usurpation, by which a subordinate group improves its position at the expense of a dominant group; and exclu-sion, by which power is maintained by exercising control downward over subordinate others. A second alternative approach arose from the Marxist view of professions. This school of thought focuses on the relations of production and the position of the professionals within the wider social structures (Navarro 1978).

The taxonomic, neo-Weberian and Marxist schools have all been critiqued. The main concern is the lack of empirical evidence to support the theories. Saks suggests that we need to investigate the explanation for state involvement in supporting strategies of professionalization; the role of specialized knowledge in securing and maintaining professional status; and the extent to which an altruistic orientation distinguishes professions from occupations. In this chapter, we shall be addressing the first two points directly, through our literature review and the presentation of empirical data.

6.2   Power, professional jurisdiction, and the State

Critical to the examination of the effect of professional boundaries is an understanding of how boundaries were, and are, established and maintained. Here the historical perspective, briefly alluded to in the introduction, is particularly helpful in understanding the foundations of the powerful position of the 'older' professions of law and medicine. Nevertheless, one cannot understand the current situation without an analysis of the relationship between the professions and the State today. Other occupations outside medicine have organized transparent systems of training and accreditation and may have widespread acceptance by the public, but these credentials do not enable the majority of them to acquire state support for independent practice. By upholding and supporting professional boundaries and jurisdictions, the State confers or supports the status and power of given professions over other occupations and groups. This differentiation has a profound effect on the health care sector.

In Freidson's early and influential work (1970), he put forward the argument that the dominance of the medical profession was dependent on the maintenance of technical autonomy, within state 'shelter'. He also made a major contribution in this early work in delineating the types of professional autonomy. In analysing the development of the profession, he underlined that the foundation of medicine's control over its work was clearly political in character. Autonomy, he suggested, was the test of professional status (Freidson 1970: 137). Freidson's recent work (2001) argues that professionalism offers a third and different logic of organizing, when compared with hierarchies or markets, and one which is entirely appropriate to specialized work. He proposes the argument that monopoly is essential to professionalism and this directly opposes it to the logic of competition in a free market. He extends this argument to suggest that monopoly and credentialism are the key elements of professionalism's economic privilege.

Johnson (1995) provides an interesting revision of ideas about the relationship between professions and the State. Drawing on the Foucaldian concept of governmentality, which views the State as a collection of institutions, procedures, tactics, knowledge, and technologies, he rejects the idea of the State as coherent and calculating. He argues that the State is not acting in a calculating way to continuously extend its apparatus of control, whilst the professions act to maximize autonomy. Rather the professions can be seen as one part of the transformation of power associated with governmentality. For Johnson, modern professions emerged as part of the apparatus that constitutes the State.

An alternative, but similar, proposal put forward by Light (1995) is that the relationship between the State and professions can be perceived as a set of countervailing powers. When power swings too profoundly towards one side or the other, it creates a countervailing backlash. He argues that the Thatcherite reforms in the UK are seen as a response to an overpowerful set of professions.

Larkin (1995) points to the need to analyse the links between inter-occupational dominance and state formation more closely. His earlier work (1983) discusses the way state and medical power converge to produce the subordination of other occupational groups within the orthodox division of labour in health care. This trend, he argues, continues. He cites the cases of the rejection of the Herbalists' Councils' attempts in the 1920s and 1930s to gain accredited training and registration and the British Medical Association's opposition to osteopaths, despite apparent acceptance (King's Fund 1991) that a cohesive body of knowledge underpinned osteopathic practice. Saks (2003) demonstrates that currently the position of the numerous types of alternative medicine is dictated by political as much as rational influences. Chiropractors are perceived to have succeeded in gaining accreditation only because of massive use by the public of this therapy.

In the UK, the professionalization project for nursing led to a long campaign by the nursing profession for a degree-based training for nurses and the removal of the grade of Enrolled Nurse (Francis and Humphreys 1999). This was an attempt to maintain exclusivity and to move from tacit/skill-based knowledge towards codified knowledge (Ainley 1994). But as Francis and Humphreys argue, this has not prevented the growth in employment of health care assistants and other less qualified staff in health care. It is also argued that raising the qualification level has priced nurses out of organizations. Currently, similar arguments are being used to suggest that nurse practitioners are being substituted for higher-priced doctors.

6.3 The role of knowledge in securing and maintaining professional status

Abbott (1988) proposes that the critical factor determining the history and development of professions is the competitive struggle between occupations for jurisdiction over areas of expertise. This shifts attention to a consideration of professions and their interaction with other occupational groups within a societal context. According to Abbott's analysis, established professions with institutionalized expertise can be understood as having achieved the end point of this competitive, political process. The foundation of Abbott's case is that a profession has its origins in negotiated jurisdictions in the workplace, which are then generalized through the establishment of such claims in the public arena and then by legal order. However, this view undervalues the ambiguity of knowledge itself and the interplay between the uncertainties of knowledge claims and political and social forces (Waddington 1973).

In a special issue in the *Journal of Management Studies*, the meaning of 'knowledge', 'knowledge work', and the 'knowledge society' was explored (Blackler et al. 1993), and in this issue, Blackler highlights the fragile, politicized, and rhetorical nature of knowledge itself. He attacks the idea of knowledge as 'objective truth' and argues against the notion of knowledge as an objective, portable, and manageable commodity. Boisot (1998) develops a robust case for a reconceptualization of knowledge and of knowledge assets within organizations. Similarly to other authors, he underlines that technological change has created new processes of knowledge production and diffusion (and that the implications of these changes are significant). He discusses the concepts of codification and abstraction. Codification is defined as a process of giving form to phenomena or experience. He argues that one could build a continuum of codification from the easy to the almost insuperable (and therefore tacit).

Scarbrough (1995) advocates a broadening of our terms towards adopting the concept of expertise, thus subsuming the term profession. The professional version of expertise focuses on the central importance of task uncertainty to the organization of knowledge-based work. His critique proposes that expertise is a more inclusive and dynamic concept. It sees knowledge as a contingent and socially distributed phenomenon, as transdisciplinary, and as associated with the economic performance of organizations. Thus expertise is a form of work that creates value through knowledge.

Establishing a claim over relevant knowledge is not sufficient to enable any group to either gain exclusive control or acknowledge State-supported professional status. Despite a long history and the widespread acceptance of nursing as a regulated and accredited profession in the UK, it has not been able to negotiate with the State for exclusive rights to a defined area of knowledge. These ongoing disputes suggest that a knowledge base cannot easily be established and verified and that the negotiation of acceptance by other groups is a highly political and competitive process. There is little evidence to suggest that the State is willing to cede power and control to 'newer' groups of experts.

This reassessment suggests the need for a more dynamic definition of expert knowledge than is provided in orthodox definitions of 'profession'. The debate so far leaves the reader with ideas to consider: To what extent is codified knowledge accepted as the sole form of 'legitimate' knowledge? In terms of the EBHC movement, to what extent is legitimate knowledge based on a medical definition and less influenced by other clinical professions/occupations? Another important question, which is explored in the next section, is: To what extent do different professionals' cognitive frameworks aid or impede the diffusion of ideas and innovations?

6.4 Becoming a professional: professional socialization and training

For the individual, the process of entering a profession and, in particular, the training undertaken may have a profound and long-lasting effect. Of special interest is the differing socialization processes involved in becoming a member of a particular profession, but the paucity of comparative research creates difficulties in exploring this issue. As a result, this section discusses uniprofessional studies that display interprofessional attitudes.

One of the most significant early texts (Etzioni 1969) clearly positions the comparative study of occupations and professions as the study of 'societal sources of tension, adaptations and their limitations'. Etzioni identifies a number of points that remain important today. Firstly, he argues that any comparative study of the health professions and occupational groups must underline that self-identity as a member of a profession means that hierarchical or organizational controls are complex and entangled with aspects of collegial control. Secondly, gender complicates the analysis. Finally, he suggests that class, family, and educational background remained (at that point) as major influencing factors of the choice of career and the entry into specific professions.

The relationship between nurses and doctors is a central one in the delivery of health care and it is, therefore, pertinent to focus discussion on this relationship. Etzioni identifies that, at the time of writing (1969), nurses and doctors were in a relationship that often prescribed who was the 'guardian' of the knowledge of the patient. Doctors were perceived to limit nurses' knowledge in various ways. This socialization process revolved around teaching nurses from whom they should get knowledge (i.e. from the doctor) and a non-questioning acceptance of instructions from the doctors. Nurses provided the tender loving care, doctors provided the 'science'. He argued that nurses and doctors were enclosed in a caste system, not a continuum of occupations.

Turner (1987) suggests that the nursing discourses of 'compliance' and 'complaint' are part of the acquisition and socialization into a subcultural occupational ideology about what the job of nursing is about. In the recent past, one of the major changes in the professionalization process for nursing occurred with the introduction of Project 2000 (UKCC 1987), which introduced radical alterations to the system of nurse training and made it a university-based education process. There was now to be a single point of entry to nurse training and the grade of Enrolled Nurse was abolished. The impetus behind these changes was an attempt to redefine the role of nursing and to conceptualize nursing as a process rather than a separate set of activities. These ideas were first introduced by Hall in 1955 and a more widespread acceptance of the concept developed in the USA, but it was not until the 1970s that it was adopted in the UK (Allen 2001). In an effort to widen the jurisdiction of nursing from purely biological functions, the 'new nursing', as it was labelled, suggested that nursing was a therapy, in which patients had to be treated holistically. Thus the notion of therapeutic communication was central to Hall's thinking.

Rafferty (1992) analyses why this programme of reform succeeded, given past failures. She suggests its success was due to a combination of nurse-driven policy changes synchronized with organizational and policy concerns. These changes have created tensions in the current health care scene. Whilst the concepts were designed to improve education and create functional autonomy, they demonstrated a lack of reality. For example, close personal relationships between individual patient and nurse are at odds with the organization of resources and their allocation in hospital and community settings. It also requires a substantial number of qualified staff, when in reality there are shortages. Commentators continue to underline the gap between nursing theory and nursing practice (Melia 1987; Allen and Hughes 2002). In addition, the individualization of care and the documentation of that process has enabled managers to exert a greater degree of external control through standard setting. Finally, the inception of an alternative qualification for support workers could be seen as providing an alternative, competing level of skilled staff. But the professionalization process continues. The recent extension of the scope of professional nursing practice (UKCC 1992) and the introduction of nurse practitioners (UKCC 1999) has potentially further extended the role of the nurse. Again these changes had been supported due to the complementary pressures from the nursing profession and reducing junior doctors' hours.

So, has the upgrading of nurses' training altered the interprofessional boundaries with medicine and other professions? An updated view of the relationships between doctors and nurses is provided by Wicks' study (1998), in which she states what the impetus for her work was:

I was nonplussed by the patronising and disrespectful attitudes of many doctors to nurses.

The study provides a number of interesting insights into the socialization processes of nurses and their work position. On the positive side, she argues that the 'gloomy' image of nursing sometimes presented in the press is mainly inaccurate and most nurses express pleasure in their work. But her study data do demonstrate that medical power continues to be imposed on both nurses and, interestingly, patients. Actions by doctors include the restriction of nursing activities, in ways which inhibit good patient care. For example, nurses were not permitted to put up blood or replace intravenous fluid with blood, but had to 'page' a doctor to come and do this. However, there are examples of work officially moving across the boundaries from doctors to nurses. Finally, a range of conflicts are displayed, with doctors and with other professionals in the workplace.

Allen's study (2001) also illuminates this question. Firstly, in discussing the relationships between doctors and nurses, her findings conclude that there are key differences at institutional and ward levels. At the level of the Trust, there is 'sustained negotiation and jurisdictional dispute in hospital management arenas'. However, at ward level, a realignment of doctors and nurses' roles appears to be taking place, with minimal negotiative effort and little conflict. The data illustrate that nurse managers had taken charge of implementing nurse role development, apparently for fear that, otherwise, medical colleagues would control the process. Certain clinical tasks were being devolved from doctors to nurses.

Whilst the studies quoted offer useful insights, there is a thin research base upon which to draw any conclusions concerning the current situation with regard to the way socialization processes affect attitudes. Nor is it possible to judge the extent to which there is greater flexibility and movement across professional boundaries. As pointed out earlier, comparative studies on other health professions are notably lacking. A recent HEFCE report (2001) underlines this. It illustrates the minute proportions of the total research budgets, which are committed to research by the nursing and allied health professions. For example, research in nursing and allied health professions received £12 million, by comparison with a total research budget of about £66 million spent on education research. The impact of a continuing uniprofessional approach to training continues to have a profound effect, which is likely to persist for some years yet. Whilst there are small-scale changes in interdisciplinary undergraduate training (Reeves and Freeth 2002), these are few in number and affect only a minority of current trainees. Multiprofessional approaches can be perceived as a threat (Cohen 2003).

There is limited evidence of any alteration in the overall power hierarchy of doctors, nurses, and allied health professionals (AHPs) at institutional level, though this is under active debate. However, at the workface, where care has to be delivered and the pressures of demand and resource shortages are most keenly felt, there is some evidence of genuine movement, with tasks moving across professional boundaries.

Being trained to behave in a 'professional' manner has been depicted as a wholly positive process of learning ethical standards and encouraging altruistic motives. But becoming a member of a profession, including accepting and adopting a set of norms and a way of behaving within an organization, is frequently learnt vicariously (Elston 1991; Walby et al. 1994; Brock et al. 1999). This can create a situation of personal conflict (Wicks 1998). There is evidence too that group norms may be stronger than ethical standards, in situations of complexity and ambiguity (Bristol Royal Infirmary Enquiry 2001).

6.5 Professionals as managers and managers as professionals

The current social and political context in which we are considering the boundaries between the health care professions in the UK is one in which the advent of new public management (NPM) has promoted a greater role for management and for management systems. It is important to note that these changes are extensive and have occurred throughout all parts of the public sector and not solely in health care. Ferlie et al. (1996) argue that the term 'new public management' encompasses both a range of characteristics, with little common agreement between authors using the term, and a series of waves of change, occurring over time. Each of these waves, it can be argued, has a differing range of priorities. Debate continues as to the extent to which one can state empirically that there has been a substantial process of 'managerialization' (Osbourne and Gaebler 1992; Ferlie et al. 1996; Hoggett 1996). The changes have led to both gains and losses in position and status for the medical profession vis-à-vis managers and other professions. Because of the successive waves of organizational change, it remains difficult to estimate the current balance of power.

Within health care, one critical issue in debates about interprofessional power is who should take decisions with major resource implications? Given that many such decisions are clinical decisions, should they be taken by clinical professionals turned managers, that is 'hybrids', or by general managers? Raising such questions highlights an immediate link to the processes of the diffusion of innovations. Decisions about the adoption of innovations, however well supported by science, are almost always influenced by cost priorities. Indeed much of the controversy concerns cost–benefit analysis. These debates, in their turn, link to changed social attitudes towards the public sector and professional services. The public adopts a more demanding attitude towards the need for transparency and visibility in management processes and service standards. The public's faith in the credibility of professionals has been shaken and clients' responses are now more questioning.

6.5.1 *Professionals as managers*

To date, much of the literature on clinical management has focused on the perceived adversarial relations of professionals versus managers. There has been a fundamental shift towards the inclusion of clinical personnel in key management roles in health care in the UK. A turning point occurred when the National Health Service (NHS) and Community Care Act (1990) introduced key structural changes with the creation of the quasi-market and the separation of purchasers and providers. This induced the need for a definable, bounded organizational service/unit as the basis of the contract. Acute and community trusts were restructured into clinical directorates virtually overnight (Fitzgerald and Sturt 1992). Montgomery (1990) drew attention to the fact that such a change can be seen either as a defensive move, to keep the voice of the collective medical profession at the forefront, or an opportunistic move, to create prestigious new employment opportunities. Despite a change of government in the UK and the altered policy agenda in health care, the trend to more clinical managers has not been reversed, but rather extended into primary care.

Significantly, limited research has been done on this trend in the UK and there are no precise figures to substantiate the number of clinicians holding posts as clinical directors of a service or as medical directors of a trust. Further substantial changes are now occurring with the establishment of Primary Care Trusts, in which general practitioners (GPs) will, for the first time, hold strategic management roles in primary care. Similar, but better documented, trends have occurred in the USA. Montgomery (1990) provides a useful analysis of the underlying conditions, which have facilitated the growth of medical managers in the USA. These conditions include the growth of larger and more complex organizations, the role of commissioners of services, and the call for greater monitoring of costs and performance standards. All of these conditions can be seen to pertain in the UK, though in differing forms. In addition, in the UK, there has been a significant shift in social trends (British Social Attitudes 2003) and several high-profile cases, which have contributed to a decrease in the public's confidence in the medical professions.

The data from recent work in the UK display a set of interrelated (and largely unresolved) issues. Firstly, there is widespread concern that the technical autonomy granted to the individual practitioner and professional systems of self-regulation have led to problems with the quality of output (Fitzgerald and Ferlie 2000; Coulter 2002).

Secondly, the movement of doctors into management roles has highlighted the tensions between professional responsibility to the individual patient and managerial responsibility to the population, in a resource-constrained system (Fitzgerald 1994; Dopson 1996). Evidence suggests that doctors display similar responses and feelings of concern when dealing with complex and uncertain changes in organizational contexts in different countries (Fitzgerald 1994; Denis et al. 1996; Hoff and McCaffrey 1996).

Finally, the employment of clinical professionals as managers and the development of clinical professional 'hybrids' raise questions concerning the effective management of professionals. What are the appropriate and effective methods for the management of clinical professionals and indeed other forms of experts? If professions have traditionally been characterized by self-regulation, can clinical professional work be improved by hybrid clinical managers, or would general managers have greater expertise and impact? To date, the evidence remains sparse. The management of professional performance is seen as the province of the members of the profession and external scrutiny is resisted. There is some evidence to illustrate that clinical managers can attack performance problems more accurately than general managers (Montgomery 1990; Fitzgerald and Dufour 1997; Kitchener 1999).

One important finding from a range of current research (Dopson 1993; Ferlie et al. 1996; Marnoch 1996) illustrates the link between professional credibility and professional knowledge. Clinical managers were strongly of the opinion that they needed to maintain their clinical practice to retain credibility with colleagues, hence the role of clinical manager is predominantly part-time. A complementary reason for this is the perceived status difference between managers and doctors. Management is still widely perceived as lower in status and 'easy' to learn.

It is evident that concomitant with the rise in clinical managers there is an increase in the range of external controls being imposed on the public sector, including health care. The advent of greater external control leads to a response from clinical professionals—'better internal controls than external controls'. Clinical managers, it can be argued, are a form of self-regulation (Fitzgerald and Ferlie 2000). Within the research on the current changes in health care in the UK, there is ample evidence to suggest that external control of complex and individualized, professional services is a difficult task. The negative response of many professionals to control systems is at least partly accounted for by the inappropriate and dysfunctional nature of the controls. A thorough review of the issues is provided by Pettigrew et al. (1999).

These trends towards a growing number of clinical managers and the implementation of managerial systems of quality monitoring with greater transparency on quality standards have fundamental implications for the career of EBHC initiatives. Firstly, we refer to our initial question posed at the start of this section: who takes the decisions? Defining the relative roles and responsibilities of clinical managers and general managers for decisions about the adoption of innovations is crucial. Furthermore, the balance of power between clinical hybrid managers and general managers is also likely to have a major influence on decisions, especially at a local level. The differing orientation and training of clinical professionals compared with general managers means that they will probably weigh the advantages and disadvantages of an innovation according to varied criteria.

Secondly, the changing nature of organizational roles may create ambiguity about role boundaries (Cassel 1997). This will require attention to issues of communication and effort to develop shared understanding about organizational (and national) priorities and the criteria for assessing 'effective' performance.

Thirdly, the trends characterized as NPM generate important questions about accountability for both individual decisions about individual patients and for systems of improvement and monitoring. If the service requires EBHC, in which innovations are adopted and used, who is responsible for ensuring this, doctors or managers? How can the patient and the public be assured that clinical staff are up to date?

We move now from this consideration of the literature to the presentation of our empirical data on professions as an aspect of context, and the impact of professional boundaries on the processes of diffusion.

6.6 Review of our empirical material on professional boundaries and their impact on translation processes

Here we suggest that the boundedness between professions and also between local 'communities of practice' inhibits the diffusion of innovations. The subtle influences and the interplay between different forms of 'boundedness' have to be analysed at multiple levels to be understood; the boundaries of the professions influence actions at national and institutional levels, but it is important to note that clin-

ical practice occurs in smaller, local groups of communities of practice, which were discussed in Chapter 2. We need to recognize that the
existence of multiple boundaries—organizational, professional, occupational, and local—create complex configurations, which are an
important aspect of the health care context.

In all of our research projects, attention is drawn to the general,
pervasive influence of professionals on the innovation diffusion.
Below is a typical report conclusion:

Despite the increased marketisation and managerialisation evident in the
health care system, professionals and their networks of information and
juridical influence have proved remarkably resilient. Local clinician 'buy-
in' is essential if national policy is not to remain abstract and underused.
(Project Acute)

6.6.1 *The role of the State in the diffusion of innovations*

The core focus of our research projects was on the processes of
diffusion of innovations. Respondents were never asked any direct
questions about their relationships with the State or with intermediate
bodies, such as the Royal Colleges. However, respondents sometimes
commented on the State's policies on health care and their impact.
The role of the State, therefore, operates indirectly in relation to the
diffusion of innovation because for many professional groups, their
professional bodies have the agency power to set and uphold quality
in the clinical standards of care. The state intervenes via legislation to
influence standards, for example, through the introduction of clinical
governance systems

6.6.2 *Professional socialization and the diffusion of innovations across social boundaries*

In discussing boundaries, we focus not primarily on the physical,
geographic, or formal boundaries between organizations, nor on the
boundaries of a single profession, but on the underpinning social and
cognitive 'boundaries' that membership of a profession creates in
relation to other professions/occupations involved in innovation
spread. We see a 'boundary' as a relatively impermeable frontier
between different occupational groups that impacts on the spread of
new work practices.

The following quote, typical in the studies, illustrates the importance of professional peers as an influence on clinical practice:

What makes me change—it's not scientific, but when I know what my peers are doing. We meet, we talk, we look at publications. (Project WNDP, consultant)

Social boundaries are created between professions and occupations by the systems of training and post-experience learning, which, as argued earlier, are largely uniprofessional. It is evident that there are considerable differences in the nature of training and level of postgraduate study, by profession. In addition to the actual differences in their specialist knowledge bases, members of a profession are taught attitudes and norms that become well embedded at an early stage in a career. Our data suggest that many health care professionals hold attitudes that are 'bounded' by the profession to which they belong.

They've been taught there is one right way to do something, and it can be difficult to get them to change. We (doctors) haven't been taught there is one right way, but only that you action what is the best evidence at the time, so we are trained to change more. (Project WNDP, doctor)

In many settings, these attitudes go unchallenged as the basic, inherited routines of health care professionals inhibit the development of a shared understanding. Building on a foundation of basic, uniprofessional training, there has also been a lack of development of routine forums for multiprofessional training in continuous professional development (CPD). This exacerbates the bounded and embedded views. Throughout the projects, these views were frequently expressed and a range of examples are given below:

Surgical decisions are almost exclusively surgeon—usually consultant— centred. That is to say, a professional colleague from a non-surgical area would have only limited decision-making power—usually only where the two disciplines overlap. (Project Acute, consultant)

A general finding from Project AC/PC was:

The self-described model of clinicians' practice is dominated by notions of individual autonomy and emergent learning.

We had a Steering group made up of largely medical opinion leaders, yet the work was done by practice nurses, who weren't involved. It did get sorted out, but it was a problem. (Project WNDP, project leader)

At the heart of many of these issues, of course, lies the differential power of the various professions. The medical profession maintains a dominant position and, in some instances, the problems are simply due to inertia or a historical unwillingness to share power.

There's a reluctance to accept that the agenda is still influenced and set by doctors. You must acknowledge that or you won't have the influence you hoped for. (Project WNDP, project leader).

Despite the influence of professional boundaries on the career of EBHC initiatives, there is ample evidence that the enrolment of multiple professional groups is an essential element of effective diffusion processes. The data illustrate the complexity of these processes and the inherent difficulties of communicating simultaneously with multiple social groups.

It doesn't matter how strong the evidence is—unless the peer group will take their colleagues in hand (and they won't), there's no mechanism to require people to abide by it. (Project PACE, doctor)

Nurses and practice managers and the CHC [Community Health Council] got left out. We were slightly scared about involving them in deference to other groups. Maybe we wrongly ascribed more value to GPs. We did consciously make a decision not to involve them. We didn't know how well the groups would mix. (Project PACE, project manager)

We didn't get the doctors on board and actively involved, because it was seen as a nursing issue and always will be. (Project WNDP, project manager)

They (the HA) don't think physiotherapy is a very effective way to spend money. Patients like it and it keeps them amused while they get better. (Project PC, GP)

This last quotation exemplifies both the stereotyping of the work and the contribution of the professions allied to medicine as 'less worthwhile', and the rather supercilious view of patients held by the speaker, a GP.

Our data are derived from examination of the micro level behaviour of individuals and groups as they interpret and enact research findings in a variety of health care contexts. It appears that such research evidence does not readily travel across professional boundaries, but in fact is 'sticky' at boundaries. Previous research (Van de Ven et al. 1999) has underlined the significance of organizational boundaries in diffusion. We suggest that strong social boundaries exist that are derived from defined professional roles and identities and reinforced by traditional work practices. To explain this behaviour, our initial analysis built on the notion that in health care, research and the adoption or acceptance of an innovation are frequently discussed within a uniprofessional 'community of practice' (Brown and Duguid 1991; Wenger 1998). Here the norm is daily, high levels of interaction. However, we found that these communities of practice have features that are different from those in non-professional contexts. These features are the largely uniprofessional nature of the community of practice; the fact that communities are typically 'self-sealing', that is they seal themselves off from neighbouring communities and defend jurisdictions; and finally, the observation that these communities are highly institutionalized.

Several critical themes emerge from this section of the analysis. Most obviously, because so many areas of care require the involvement of more than one profession for the diffusion of an innovation, it frequently requires the active involvement of people from many professional groups, and the diffusion process has to find ways across these social barriers. These contextual variations in interrelationships can have a profound effect on the outcome and whether change or improvement can be implemented. Projects PACE and WNDP focused on pilot projects and demonstration sites that attracted specific funding. As a consequence, they examined the role of project management in facilitating the diffusion of the innovations. Many project managers recognized or learnt that it was essential to complete a stakeholder analysis in order to identify and plan for the different groups involved.

In explaining and accounting for the variations in the rate of diffusion between sites and between cases, several of our studies underline the critical importance of traversing professional boundaries and gaining agreement from, or developing joint approaches to, the implementation of innovations. However, this can only be achieved if a reasonable foundation of interprofessional relations already exists.

The creation of trusting working relationships is very important. Relationships provide the conduit to achieve change. (Project WNDP, project manager)

Where this is not the case, it is probable that only limited progress can be made. Within our studies, examples exist of both positive interrelationships, where substantial change had been implemented:

I think most of my colleagues in the department are happy to work in a multidisciplinary way. I trust the midwives. You have to be available; have to give feedback to people to be counted on. We have a stable senior midwifery group in this hospital. (Project Acute, consultant) and negative interrelationships, where very limited progress had occurred:

I suppose the main sweeping change has been the less active participation in pregnancy care by consultant obstetricians and more active involvement by other colleagues, namely the GPs and the midwives apparently. . . . I have no idea how actively involved they are, they tell me they are and since they are accountable to themselves, they are their own masters. They have not invited me to comment, so then I believe them. (Project Acute, consultant)

There is considerable supporting evidence of the continued dominance of the medical profession within the clinical setting, particularly in the processes adopted to draw up clinical protocols and guidelines. These processes are almost universally led by doctors and, in some settings, all decisions are taken by doctors without even consultation with other professionals. There is also a clear structural reinforcement of the dominant medical position, in that many managerial/leadership roles are held by doctors.

6.6.3 *Cognitive professional boundaries and hierarchies of credible evidence*

In this section, we develop our analysis further to suggest that in addition to social boundaries, the diffusion of innovations is also impeded by the presence of cognitive or epistemological boundaries. One further consequence of differing training and socialization processes is the existence of hierarchies of evidence. In our data, we found differences of view expressed by GPs and acute hospital consultants/doctors, the two largest groups of interviewees in these studies as to the nature of the hierarchy of evidence. GPs were much more likely to question the relevance of the randomized controlled trial (RCT) as a 'gold' standard for good research. They held a broader view of the criteria for diagnostic and treatment decisions and weighed the scientific evidence differently, against the social and psychological aspects of the whole patient. These differential views are accentuated, because it is apparent that in many instances there is no clear, definitive evidence, a point we look at in-depth in Chapter 7.

In fact, there were doubts about the evidence in all cases, more so in some than in others. (Project WNDP, report conclusions)

General concerns about RCTs amongst GPs were exacerbated by the additional problems seen to relate to primary care.

[T]hat is the one big problem with primary care evidence-based medicine at the moment, that is that most of the evidence we are encouraging GPs to change their behaviour on is actually very much secondary care based. (Project PC, GP educator)

Nurses and, to a lesser extent, midwives were more likely to admit that they expected to follow the instructions of the consultant and not necessarily inspect the source of the evidence themselves. But many nurses and midwives argued the need to adopt a holistic view of the patient; they were more questioning of the gaps in the research base and the lack of interest in the 'routine' case.

A number of interviewees reported (Project PC) that in their experience nurses 'have a more receptive culture to clinical effectiveness', and 'are much better at following a template of care' than doctors, even though there is less research evidence about nursing.

Midwives exemplify a professional group, which is increasingly interested in the evidence base and consequentially more questioning in their attitudes.

Research has shown that CTGs [cardiotocograms] have not brought down the mortality rate. It is not particularly efficacious; all the research shows that there are no real benefits in using a monitor provided the midwife is well qualified. (Project Acute, midwife)

Therapists accept that the research base for their care is underexplored and recognize the need to conduct more investigation. The low research tradition, coupled with shortage of funding and the competition with doctors for research funding, are seen as enduring problems. Some therapists put forward interesting arguments about whether 'therapy' is susceptible to the RCT approach.

I would say that primary care is the 'tail end Charlie'. And the research that has been done does not stand up to critical appraisal. If you think that it is all pretty soft—we are usually involved with mixed methodologies—it is very hard to completely isolate therapy from the rest. And so there are some concerns that if we go down the path of gold standard studies and we all do blind control studies that you will actually destroy what therapy is anyway. (Project PC, physiotherapist)

Some of the differences of view may be explained by the differential skills that group members have to enable them to access and interpret the research base. On other occasions, these differences might be seen as part of wider controversies and disputes about an approach to, or regime of, care.

Whereas the methodology of our studies did not include the collection of data directly from users, there were also indications that users' views of credible evidence may be based on a wider or differing set of criteria from those of medical/clinical staff. One distinction appears to be that users take into account the experience of the condition, the pain or discomfort involved, and the extent of its impact on daily life. Thus, credible evidence was any evidence that provided data on how to ameliorate the condition, whatever its source. Users perceived long-term and non-life-threatening conditions that create pain to be of higher importance than did clinicians. Medical staff, especially specialist staff, focus on criteria that give primacy to life-threatening conditions. This may account for the mass movement of patients towards the use of alternative medicine, which has offered care for conditions such as back pain.

Overall, these data suggest that to understand diffusion processes we need to recognize that cognitive boundaries exist between and within health care professions. Knowledge is often held within professional boundaries, so that the knowledge base claimed by a profession and its traditions of thought are closely intertwined. These differing knowledge bases and traditions create cognitive boundaries. The evidence or knowledge underpinning the innovations did not readily flow across the professions; rather it often stuck. Professions display different research cultures, agendas, and questions. The barriers have a cognitive as well as a social or identity-based element. These cognitive boundaries operate in combination with the social group boundaries to form the complex social context that influences the career of EBHC innovations.

6.6.4 *Mechanisms for moving across boundaries*

In discussions of the so-called 'implementation gap,' much attention has centred on the question of access to evidence and to a research database, and less on the means by which evidence can be debated and consensus reached at local level, within and between the communities of practice.

It is apparent that implementation strategies occurred more frequently in those researches that studied 'pilot' projects (Projects GR and PACE) and national development projects (Project WNDP), than in the projects that followed the natural career of an innovation. The second case study in Project Acute represents an interesting example of a strategy that can be characterized as a mixture of nationally led, 'top-down' intervention and local engagement, with the national initiative on 'Changing Childbirth' seen as a main influence:

The watershed and the crystallisation of the way things were going was the 'Changing Childbirth' document itself. And I think the units which were being innovative and moving forward put much greater emphasis on midwifery group practices, continuity of care for the woman both antenatally and through labour and delivery. (Project Acute, midwife)

However, it is notable that appropriate forums for sharing and debating evidence locally are lacking or poorly integrated into organizational and clinical routines.

There isn't a mechanism to translate the experience into a learning set. The hospital managers aren't involved or accountable. (Project WNDP, project manager)

There are some rare examples of 'bridging' roles that demonstrate the benefits of active facilitation in encouraging the sharing of evidence across professional boundaries. Such roles include the clinical role of the research midwife and the managerial role of the project leader or facilitator. It is apparent that without active facilitation, the timescale for developing shared learning and changed perceptions is significant.

There are also some rare examples of regular forums for sharing and debating evidence interprofessionally. In Project PC, one of the studies featured a general practice with a range of regular meetings and forums for interprofessional exchange which were well attended. In this context, one respondent described the organization:

I think we are very team orientated and I think we recognize the other members of the team far more than other places do and encourage them to develop their own skills and interests. (Project PC, GP)

The development of such forums is delayed by the apparent existence of formal interprofessional forums, which often are not authentic. Across the studies, examples of these occurred in all sectors of health care and included GP practice meetings and audit meetings in acute hospitals. Many such meetings are not well attended by all the affected professions and subsequently there are low levels of interaction. This is sometimes explained as 'lack of interest by the nurses', but without any apparent understanding of how one facilitates a genuine interaction.

Chapter 5 referred to the critically important role that is played by opinion leaders in the health care context. In considering here the mechanisms which may be used to facilitate sharing of knowledge across boundaries, we remind the reader of the vital role that opinion leaders can play and the need for skilled strategic leadership in this area. We revisit this point in Chapter 8.

6.6.5   *The role of professionals as managers*

We have postulated that the boundaries between the various health care professions are often 'sealed'. However, the gulf between the worlds of clinical professionals and others, particularly between doctors and managers, is, it appears, even greater. Innovation and clinical change is still seen, in the main, as the sole domain of the clinical professional. As we mentioned in Chapter 5, throughout these projects, managers were distant figures in the innovation processes we studied.

In Project AC/PC, a useful summary of the key influences on clinical decisions is produced and is provided here for reference as Table 6.1.

This provides an overview of the low level of influence exerted by general managers. Acute sector respondents did not rate managers as an influence at all, whilst amongst primary care sector respondents between 78 and 89 per cent rated managers' influence as 'low'.

In a number of the projects, there was some limited recognition of the need for project management and for other managerial skills to secure changes in practice.

Projects like this are very tender flowers; they require protecting and nurturing by a senior health authority figure—it ought to be the CEO or at least the DPH. (Project WNDP, Director of Public Health)

You certainly need your clinical champions, but you also need public health and/or managers involved as well, because the clinicians don't always have the knowledge of what you need to get things through the system, how to work the management structure. (Project PACE, project manager)

6.7   Concluding remarks

6.7.1   *On the power of the professions and power dynamics within the diffusion process*

Throughout these data, one consistent theme across all of the projects is the critical importance of the professions in the diffusion of innovations.

Knowledge to Action?

Table 6.1 *Comparison of influences on practice for asthma and glue ear*

	Asthma (% of respondents)	Glue ear (% of respondents)
High importance		
Clinical experience	85	69
Royal Colleges/BTS guidelines	78	
Ongoing training	73	57
Patient/Parental views		60
Hospital colleagues		53
(Primary care respondents only)		
Local guidelines	51	51
Other consultants in Trust	51	
Low importance		
Market/Competition	88	96
Referring GPs	84	68
Contract specifications	81	74
Mass media	71	79
Health authority managers		78
Financial considerations	67	74
Patient pressure groups	66	
Drugs reps	64	
Your own research	60	65
Risk of litigation	55	74
PHCT	54	
Pharmacists	53	
Local colleagues outside Trust		55
Effective Health Care Bulletin		54
Nurses/Health visitors		50

Most frequently mentioned 'high importance' and 'low importance' from tick lists.

When considering the transfer of innovations and ideas across organizations and across professional groups in health care, it is apparent that individual professionals and professional groups (particularly the doctors) have the power to impede or to facilitate diffusion processes. The consequences of this finding alone are critical. If the quality of health care delivery is to be improved, we need to understand the complex, historically and contextually informed interaction between different professional groups, and to design diffusion strategies that acknowledge this complexity. There is no evidence at all to support the view that managers or project managers alone could produce an intervention strategy that would generate active participation from clinicians in processes of innovation adoption. To engage clinical staff requires skilled clinical leaders and the engagement of credible members of the professions (opinion leaders) in the diffusion process.

In the discussion of the literature, we argued that to understand how occupational boundaries are maintained or expanded, we need to analyse the dynamic relationships between professional and occupational groups and the State over time. We saw that whilst there is some evidence of work moving across sectoral and professional boundaries (Richardson and Maynard 1995; Sandall 1995; Allen and Hughes 2002; Cohen 2003) as a result of innovations, generally, the historically ordered hierarchy of the health care professions appears unchanged. In our cases, there was virtually no evidence of the power of the medical profession over other health care professions being diminished. At the local level, within systems of practice, there were examples of medical groups that operate with barely any reference or consultation with other professional groups in decision-making, for example in the surgical cases. In other instances, there were signs of pressures from within the service and from outside combining to cause some reconsideration of how work was configured and who had prime responsibility; for example in asthma care, where nursing has taken more and more responsibility for the diagnosis and management of the condition. This evidence is interesting when one considers the current policy statements that highlight the need for professional boundaries to be more flexible. A sustained flow of policy documents (Cmnd 3807, 1997; DoH 1998; Cmnd 4818, 2000; DoH 2001a) has argued for fundamental shifts in the boundaries between the health care professions. These documents set out targets concerning increased responsiveness to patients, the development of integrated services and new roles, and a review of skill mix. All of these changes are aimed at improving the quality of care and reducing variations in clinical care and standards.

In line with our findings concerning the sustained system of inter-professional power relationships, we observe that these professional boundaries continue to be maintained by state support. The relationship between the State and professions is a more complex relationship than the notion of 'countervailing power' proposed by Light (1995), because not all the professions and/or the semi-professions have identical interests. The state is partially dependent on the professions for the delivery of the health service and must therefore balance the demands of the 'established' and 'establishing' professions. There are some significant indications of external pressure to tighten professional quality regulation by moving towards accreditation and reaccreditation systems. The recent move towards revalidation of doctors would be one example. However, the revalidation process, which has now been agreed (GMC 2003), will be based on 'full participation in annual appraisal, with completed supporting documentation', during the five-year cycle. Clearly this is an acceptance by the State of a process that remains within professional control. There are small shifts too in the licensing of other allied health professions, as in the case of chiropractors, but only after long campaigns. As Montgomery (1990) has previously argued, credentialling appears to provide a mechanism for maintenance of an established power position and to be a modern-day form of closure.

6.7.2   *On the changing social relationships of professional work*

Clinical professionals recount, and sometimes lament, changing relationships with patients and health care users. Many clinical staff considered that patients are more demanding and less respectful. Patients, on the other hand, may have a variety of expectations of health care providers, but a proportion suggest they expect a certain degree of 'efficient service' from the system and also more information and explanation of options and risks in treatment.

In considering the ongoing changes in the social relations of professional work and the power of the medical and clinical professions, a number of curious contradictions appear. Many professionals acknowledge that patients' expectations of professionals are changing. Professionals perceive many pressures on themselves and on their practice—they see these pressures as economically driven, as driven by increasing trends towards litigation, and as managerially driven. Many medical staff do not perceive themselves as empowered (Smith 2001; Edwards et al. 2002). Yet our data suggest the continued power of the medical profession and continued ability to enclave areas of practice. Whilst there is a downward pressure on the efficient use of expensive, skilled manpower, areas of work only appear to be given up reluctantly by one profession or occupation to another less qualified group (Rolfe et al. 1999; Allen and Hughes 2002).

6.7.3   *On the complexity of professional boundaries and influence processes*

Health care is a multiprofessional domain: the mechanisms of influence are complex and the dynamics of intra- and interprofessional relationships at any one time and in any specific location have to be understood. To comprehend and analyse organizational events, one needs to examine multilevel influences from the national, institutional, and local levels. Within this multiprofessional domain, the intra- and interprofessional interactions and the processes of influence have both static and dynamic elements to them. Our evidence illustrates that active processes of sharing and engaging professionals are required if innovations are to diffuse in health care settings. For such processes to be effective requires an understanding of the complex dynamics and the mechanisms of influence. Part of this complexity relates to the process of entry into a profession and the subsequent education and training.

Our data suggest that there were often poor informal and formal links between collocated professional communities of practice even within the same health care organization. Unlike Brown and Duguid (2001*b*), we did not find, however, that geographical proximity led to effective sharing of information. Rather it was the social and cognitive boundaries within health care that inhibited the diffusion of innovations within and between professional communities of practice. These boundaries also exist between the various clinical professional groups and managers. Therefore, to better understand the diffusion of innovations into practice, we need to refocus attention on such boundaries as a key part of the context, as these are critical and under-researched. With a larger data-set, one can reinforce the validity of findings from our prior work (Ferlie et al. 2005), that the social and cognitive boundaries within health care largely inhibit the diffusion of innovations within and between professional communities of practice. One can further extend the analysis to suggest that these boundaries also exist between the various clinical professional groups and managers and that between these particular occupations, such boundaries are even more significant.

Our data suggest that one can identify varying configurations of multiple boundaries, some of which are concrete and transparent, such as spatial, organizational boundaries, when two parts of the same organization are located five miles apart. Other boundaries are observable, but their impact may be less transparent, such as membership of different professions. Finally, there are less transparent forms of boundaries, such as social and epistemic, created by identification with a professional group. Within any given context, the more numerous and impermeable the boundaries are, the more diffusion of the innovation is inhibited.

In considering the mutually reinforcing nature of these social and epistemic boundaries, we seek to build on the work of Brown and Duguid (2001*a*) which debates how it is that knowledge manifests 'stickiness' and 'leakiness' simultaneously. They argue that sociocultural accounts offer richer explanations of these dynamics than a focus on the nature of the knowledge itself. By shifting their analysis to the practice dimensions of communities of practice, they underline the link between learning and identity. They argue that work identities are built through participation and social contact. Knowledge may diffuse within communities of practice, but stick where practice is not shared. Our empirical data support the view that social boundaries between different communities of practice and between professions and occupations are reinforced by cognitive boundaries.

A cumulative process can be seen in operation. Our current analysis suggests that the social and cognitive boundaries that exist between professions and other occupations, such as managers, can be perceived in operation at two intersecting levels. Firstly, social and epistemic boundaries of varying impact and impermeability exist between different professions, such as doctors and physiotherapists, and between clinical professionals and managers. Secondly, social and epistemic boundaries exist between the local communities of practice, which in health care are frequently uniprofessional. There was little or no evidence that communities of practice were habitually multidisciplinary. The community of practice and the professional group are also the dominant reference groups for an individual.

We suggest that within professional organizations, one finds a complex set of interactive influences on the diffusion process. Our data enable us to elucidate apparently contradictory findings from prior research reviewed earlier in this chapter. At the level of the profession or occupation, whilst our findings appear to contradict the prior literature that presents professional networks as positive facilitators (Coleman et al. 1966; Robertson et al. 1996) of innovation, we can see that such professional networks are examples of 'networks of practice' as described by Brown and Duguid. These are epistemic networks of similar practitioners that help to share learning across organizational boundaries. At the level of the local community of practice, our data concur with the findings of recent work (Swan et al. 2002), which illustrates the difficulties experienced by managers in attempting to construct communities of practice from several different medical subspecialities. Their case shows how management had to utilize networking and brokerage techniques to overcome the disciplinary barriers. This research reinforces the contention that only where epistemic cultures are shared (Knorr-Cetina 1999) will networks within and across organizations facilitate diffusion.

The data presented here illustrate that there is a cumulative impact that varies from one context to another. This negative impact accumulates from a combination of varying 'boundary' impediments, such as organizational boundaries, combined with social and cognitive boundaries. Communities of practice stimulate learning and change internally within the local group, but this group membership can impede the spread of ideas from one community to another. In explaining the varying rates and speed of diffusion in specific locations, one notes that the configuration of boundaries can accumulate, to generate more impediments in one organization than another. This underlines that to generate effective processes of innovation within any given organization, one has to focus on current work practices, the historical roots of such practices, and the extent and quality of intergroup relations. Because these inhibitors are cumulative, one needs to adopt a holistic, system perspective to analyse contexts. Research that looks at one lever and/or one group misses the accumulative effect. In health care, therefore, there may be multiple and reinforcing boundaries that impede diffusion and vary in their impermeability from case to case.

7

Knowledge, Credible Evidence, and Utilization

Louise Fitzgerald and Sue Dopson

7.1 Introduction

One starting point for understanding how new knowledge and innovations are adopted and put into use in health care is to consider the meaning of the terms 'knowledge' and 'evidence', as used in the term evidence-based health care (EBHC). How do these definitions compare? In this chapter, we shall build on the discussion presented in Chapter 3 on EBHC to consider what makes evidence credible to potential users, who are mainly members of the health care professions. Thus, necessarily, we shall link to Chapters 5 and 6, which considered the characteristics of the context of health care organizations and, more particularly, the impact of multiple professions and professional boundaries on the career of EBHC initiatives.

Rich (1997) reflects on the development of research on knowledge utilization, from the perspective of the impact on policy. He makes the point that distinctions have been drawn between the definitions of data as raw material; information as refined data, which provides added value; and knowledge, which provides added value *and* has been subjected to some validation or 'truth test'. Critically, he points out, however, that what constitutes a 'truth test' is contestable. Bell (1999) makes the point that data, information, and knowledge can be arranged on a single continuum, depending on the extent to which they reflect human involvement in, and processing of, reality. In Chapter 6, we introduced the idea proposed by Blackler (1995) that knowledge is fragile, politicized, and rhetorical in nature. He argues that there is no 'objective truth', and that knowledge is not an objective and portable commodity. Most usefully here, we draw on Tsoukas and Vladimirou's definition of knowledge (2001). This definition is especially illuminating because the authors address the question of the differences, in the first instance, between knowledge and organizational knowledge and the implications of both definitions for knowledge management. Importantly, the work seeks to conceptualize the links between knowledge and organizational action. Tsoukas and Vladimirou (2001: 974) start by posing the questions:

How is knowledge brought to bear on what an individual does? What are the prerequisites for using knowledge effectively in action?

These authors argue that 'knowledge is the individual ability to draw distinctions within a collective domain of action, based on an appreciation of context or theory, or both'. More simply, this definition tells us that though knowledge is an attribute of the individual, the ability involves distinguishing how ideas will work in social situations or the 'collective domains' where action occurs; and in order to draw the relevant distinctions, the individual requires an appreciation of either the context of action or generic theory or both. So, knowledge is not just a mental attribute. It involves individual judgement and the interaction of the individual with some potential context for action. The exercise of judgement is based on the ability of the individual to draw distinctions and locate himself or herself within a collectively generated and sustained domain of action—a 'practice'. We shall return to these ideas in the concluding section when we have considered other literature and our empirical data.

Tsoukas and Mylonopoulos (2004) also stress the socially constructed nature of knowledge. The preoccupation with the 'implementation gap' (Lomas and Haynes 1988; Mulrow 1994; West et al. 1999) has been discussed in Chapters 2 and 3. Interestingly, within this debate the precise definition of evidence is rarely contested. Evidence is seen as the given and accepted element, and attention focuses on the availability of, and access to, evidence; the ability to interpret and assess evidence; and the uptake and adoption of evidence. Within the EBHC literature, the discussion focuses on evidence, not knowledge, and it rarely distinguishes between them. There is limited cross-citation of texts and research between the debate on EBHC and the wider literature of innovation, knowledge creation, and diffusion in commercial firms.

We noted in Chapter 3 that critiques of EBHC have suggested that it places an overly rigid and reductionist emphasis on scientific evidence, as the primary determinant of clinical practice. Indeed authors such as Williamson (1992) and Hunter (1996) argue that the EBHC movement will reinforce the historical hierarchical distinction between the quantifiable and measurable facts of research as evidence and the tacit knowledge derived from clinical practice. McKee and Clarke (1995) suggest that EBHC's definition of evidence undervalues medicine's more holistic and empathic side, in which judgement, experience, and skill play an important part.

This chapter considers these competing discussions and suggests the need for more clearly agreed definitions of knowledge and evidence. Linking the two concepts, the term 'evidence', as it is used in health care, is perceived to be similar to the definition of information as refined data which provides added value, as proposed by Rich (1997). Within health care terminology there are specific connotations of the nature of acceptable information for clinical decision-making. Evidence, in these terms, is more narrowly defined. Knowledge, on the other hand, is the acceptance and application of evidence within a given context.

7.2　From knowledge creation to diffusion and management

Looking across the various literatures on knowledge creation and diffusion, the diffusion of innovations, and the so-called 'implementation gap' in EBHC, a somewhat confusing, fragmented, and sometimes contradictory picture emerges. A number of the causes of this haphazard accumulation of research data have already been reviewed in various syntheses that exist of the literature on innovation diffusion. Damanpour (1991), Wolfe (1994), and Fiol (1996) provide useful overviews of the research, and highlight the seemingly contradictory and non-cumulative aspects of the research. They also direct attention to future research agendas. These authors identify the various interlinked, but differing, foci of research, which include processes of creativity and innovation—the ideas/knowledge creation phase; processes of innovation uptake and development—the innovation prioritization and commercialization phase; and processes of innovation adoption and diffusion, both intraorganizationally and interorganizationally—the phases of uptake and spread. These phases are not separated, but there are elements of a developmental sequence (Van de Ven et al. 1999). One significant finding of these reviews is in the disproportionate attention paid to the post-knowledge creation stages. In this chapter, we attempt to rebalance this by considering the nature of the knowledge or evidence itself.

There is a considerable literature, mainly based on the private, 'for-profit' sector, which identifies new modes of knowledge production and diffusion, the commodification of knowledge, and the impact of information technology on the sharing of knowledge (Fincham et al. 1994; Gibbons et al. 1994; Blackler 1995; Scarbrough 1996; Boisot 1998). These authors argue that it is becoming harder for organizations and individuals to control knowledge assets. Yet the case has been made that knowledge and knowledge creation will be the source of competitive advantage in the developed world (Hamel and Prahalad 1994; Nonaka and Takeuchi 1995).

Nonaka et al. (2000, 2001: 14) define knowledge as 'justified true belief' with the emphasis on the 'justified' and not the 'true'. They make the argument that in Western epistemology 'truthfulness' is perceived as the essential attribute of this definition and is absolute, static, and non-human. Within their definition, however, knowledge is dynamic, created in social interactions, and is context specific. (This definition has much in common with that of Tsoukas and Vladimirou's quoted above.) Nonaka et al. (2001) emphasize the differences between explicit and tacit knowledge, seeing both as complementary to each other. The focus of their thesis is on the organizational knowledge creation process. They propose a model of knowledge creation which has three parts: the socialization, externalization, combination, and internalization (SECI) process, which converts tacit to explicit knowledge; Ba, which is the shared context of cognition and action; and leading, which involves creating the conditions for knowledge creation. Whilst each of the modes of SECI may be observed separately, they also occur in interaction, and the continuous process of knowledge creation is described as dynamic interactions forming a spiral.

Garvey and Williamson (2002) expand the definition of tacit knowledge, defining it as 'the sum total of an individual's experience, fully internalised and more than they can express'. Tacit knowledge in this definition brings together the technical/scientific and rational *and* the personal, emotional, and intuitive. As discussed in Chapter 6, authors, such as Boisot (1998), writing from a knowledge management perspective also address similar themes. Boisot develops a robust case for a reconceptualization of knowledge and of knowledge assets within organizations. He introduces the concepts of codification and abstraction. Codification is defined as a process of giving form to phenomena or experience. He argues that one could build a continuum of codification from the easy to the almost insuperable (and therefore tacit). Abstraction is the process of discerning the structures that underlie the forms. These definitions include critical understandings of the differences between tacit and formal knowledge that are poorly understood. Based on these ideas, Boisot produces a conceptual framework for understanding knowledge flows, known as I Space. This proposes that the more codified and abstract an item of information becomes, the larger the percentage of a given population it will reach in a given time. He propounds the concept of fluid and viscous knowledge. Fluid knowledge is knowledge which is well codified and abstract; all extraneous data have been shed. Viscous knowledge is data rich, qualitative, and ambiguous. It flows slowly, if at all. He makes the crucial point that knowledge assets, unlike physical assets, can be shared with others and retained at the same time. Whilst sharing the knowledge does not reduce its utility, it does reduce its value. Boisot continues by arguing that diffusability should not be confused with adoption. Conceptually, Boisot offers useful means for increasing our understanding of types of knowledge, but there is limited empirical data here to underpin these ideas on the processes of knowledge sharing and diffusion.

Further empirical data to support these concepts are available from the substantial programme of research known as the Minnesota studies (Van de Ven et al. 1999). These data demonstrate that the overall process of innovation involves many iterations and changes of prioritization and judgements, based on changing values. This dynamic is partly accounted for by the fluid involvement of different individuals and groups in various phases of the process. Sharing meanings between different individuals and groups may be a fraught and unpredictable process.

Brown and Duguid's work (1991, 2001a, 2002) offers many useful insights in this area. Brown and Duguid (2001a) confront the argument that different kinds of knowledge are either 'sticky' (i.e. tacit) or 'leaky' (i.e. explicit), arguing that this proposition does not hold good when one observes that the same knowledge may be sticky in one organization and flow or leak in another. (This is similar to Boisot's definition of viscous and fluid knowledge.) They suggest that sociocultural accounts offer richer explanations because work practice is critical to understanding the acquisition of identity and knowledge at work. The concept of 'communities of practice' (Lave and Wenger 1991) provides their unit of analysis. Examining the connection between practice and knowledge, Brown and Duguid (2001a) draw on Polanyi (1966), who concluded that explicit and tacit knowledge were *not* separate categories, but that knowledge always has a tacit *dimension*. Tacit knowledge is required to make explicit knowledge tradable and mobile. Therefore, there is a need to share some practice to be able to share new ideas. To understand where and why knowledge flows in health care (and where it does not), we need to examine the situations in which health care professionals genuinely share practice and thus develop common practices. We may also need to analyse the contextual features that facilitate this sharing. These become crucial issues in understanding and interpreting the empirical data from health care, which we shall present.

Other critics of the knowledge management literature include Garvey and Williamson (2002), who question whether it is knowledge exploitation or knowledge exploration? They critique the rationalistic basis of much management thinking and quote Von Krogh et al. (1994): 'there is no longer a right knowledge, but many coexisting conflicting pieces of knowledge.' Sense-making, they argue, is part of a knowledge-productive environment.

Thus far in our review of the knowledge management literature, the political dimensions of knowledge acquisition and of knowledge dissemination have surfaced as themes. Fincham et al. (1994) focus directly on issues of the management and control of expertise and knowledge production and diffusion. These authors argue that rationalistic explanations of innovation and diffusion ignore the political processes of interest articulation and accommodation that surround decision-making. On the basis of their data, they advocate a management of *expertise* approach, to surmount the division between the political and knowledge processes. This approach recognizes that expertise, as compared with knowledge, has several components: the knowledge itself, evaluation by communities of peers or members of a 'reputational network,' and a system that validates and rewards the knowledge claim. Knowledge, they argue, only becomes expertise after it has been evaluated by like others from within a peer or professional group. This process involves a more collective acknowledgement of the 'worth' of the knowledge. Following this acknowledgement, there will be a system that rewards the knowledge claim, as when publishing in a 'reputable' journal such as the *British Medical Journal* becomes a criterion for promotion. The evidence offered in Chapter 5 identifies the crucial role played by opinion leaders in this reputational network. In Chapter 6, we illustrated the importance of professional membership and professional boundaries to our understanding of these reputational networks and knowledge dissemination. Robertson et al. (1996) also draw attention to the critical role of professional networks and the manner in which they can be used to promote particular bodies of knowledge.

Debates about the nature of new knowledge and innovation processes drawn from outside the health care literature clearly have many implications for our understanding of the diffusion of knowledge and of the more narrowly defined 'evidence'. The full breadth of this literature has rarely informed debates about EBHC and yet we have found this work useful in dissecting the analysis of our empirical data. In the following sections, we focus on the empirical data from our projects which explores the way organizational members interpret evidence and decide on its credibility (or otherwise). Our particular interest is in the ways in which evidence is construed as valid and robust knowledge, which will be used in practice. In Chapter 8, we explore further the process of getting knowledge into practice.

7.3   Review of empirical data on the credibility of evidence

This section is divided into four: Section 7.3.1 looks at professionals' perceptions of what makes 'evidence' credible and discovers differences of view; Section 7.3.2 examines the processes involved in accepting evidence and whether these are based largely on direct appraisal of the evidence or on trust of the opinion of valued others; and Sections 7.3.3 and 7.3.4 explore beyond the boundaries of published, codified evidence to discover other sources of influence that may affect the behaviour of professionals and therefore the career of EBHC initiatives.

7.3.1   *A hierarchy of evidence? Perceptions of credible evidence*

Across all our cases, the spread pathways of innovations were slow, complex, and contested. Strong limits to spread were evident amongst the evidence-based innovations, indicating limits to 'science push'. Fieldwork frequently highlighted higher levels of innovation complexity than originally supposed. Our studies confirm non-linear models of innovation spread (Van de Ven et al. 1999). Robust science does not 'flow' into use; indeed 'flow' is a radically inappropriate image to describe erratic, circular, or abrupt processes, which may come to a full stop or go into reverse. One major reason accounting for this is the inherent difficulty of interpreting 'the evidence'.

Our data demonstrate that in many instances, scientific evidence does not appear to the beholder as clear, accepted, and bounded. There is no such thing as 'the evidence', there are simply bodies of evidence, usually competing bodies of evidence. Even the research agenda and, therefore, the available bodies of evidence are socially and historically constructed. For example, the final report of Project AC/PC states:

Respondents, including specialists—often concluded that it was difficult to discern clear messages from 'the evidence'.

There was some disagreement, but little evidence of intense controversy in asthma and glue ear.

The accounts paint a picture of clinical practice which is constrained by, or seen as acceptable within, loosely defined boundaries. We don't see controversies per se, rather there are 'grey' areas where there is no incontrovertible evidence available to resolve clinical questions.

Within Project PC, the appraisal of evidence was made even more difficult when it involved adaptation to different patient populations. In Project GR, the project on the use of steroids in preterm labour was seen to have the clearest evidence, yet:

Even where there was a 'state-of-the-art' and uncontroversial review of the evidence with clear implications for practice, its detailed application to clinical policy, let alone individual practice, proved problematic.

In the stroke care project in Project GR, it was stated:

On close examination, the available reviews were usually not systematic, rigorous, nor geared towards decisions that clinicians, rather than purchasers, would need to make.

This view was mirrored in Project WNDP:

(The review) helped to focus down on the strongest areas and be clear where it was weak.

Good evidence was necessary but not sufficient. Many interviewees commented on the importance of debate and interaction between clinical peers.

As discussed already, strong evidence could act as a 'push' factor to encourage clinicians to embark on changes to their practice. In a number of examples, individuals and project teams gained a sense of confidence from knowing that the evidence was strong enough to avoid 'having academic argument all the way through'. Where there was a will to change practice (e.g. because of perceived defects in the system, or because the clinicians were becoming aware that their practice did not match that of their opinion leaders), having a review of the evidence gave the confidence to say:

There aren't many things where the evidence is there—5–10% maybe. What [the researcher who had reviewed the literature] did was to make it very concrete and clear where there was and wasn't evidence. So where in the millions of places she said the jury was out, we were able to make sensible decisions. . . . It gave us confidence. (Project GR, consultant)

Finally, we note in Project PACE:

One of the original criteria for selecting the 16 project sites was that the work should be based on 'robust' evidence. One would, therefore, expect strong consensus from the interviews that the evidence for each project was strong and convincing. In practice, perceptions of the strength of the evidence varied both between projects and sometimes between members of the same team.

There was ambivalence about the pre-eminence of randomized controlled trials (RCTs) in the hierarchy of evidence available to inform practice. Knowing what kind of evidence would be most convincing seemed to be an important part of influencing practice. In short, RCTs, especially for doctors, were the acme of evidence in theory, but not always in practice. On the one hand, it was accepted that RCTs are *theoretically* the highest, that is most scientifically reliable, form of evidence. Systematic reviews were regarded—again in theory if not in practice—as an important source of evidence by many interviewees, although at the time in which our studies were conducted, the Cochrane collaboration was relatively young and still developing. It is worth noting, however, that there may have been a tendency for interviewees to say what they felt was expected of them, a point that was most explicitly noted in one of our studies (Project AC/PC), which asked clinicians about the sources of knowledge that they believed most influenced their clinical decisions. Thus, doctors in particular tended to respond positively to questions about the role of RCTs (which are after all a fundamental part of the paradigm that they work to as a profession).

On the other hand, despite this accepted norm that RCTs should be the most persuasive type of evidence, we found that doctors often had more respect for the tacit, experiential knowledge of respected colleagues, including non-medical health professionals, than they did for research evidence. Nevertheless, nurses and allied health professionals (AHPs) would sometimes report that they felt doctors would be more likely to listen to them if only there were more RCT-based evidence in their own professional areas.

There was much discussion about the limitations of evidence from RCTs. Our seven studies found repeated examples of doubt, scepticism, or downright cynicism about the role of RCTs in providing relevant evidence to inform everyday practice. This was the case even where the organization had selected clinical areas for improvement precisely because of the belief that clear research evidence from RCTs had not been implemented. There was a sense among many of our interviewees that they were sometimes asked to implement research evidence that, whilst ostensibly relevant, was not strictly applicable to their own practice. General practitioners (GPs), for example, would typically point out that most RCTs are done with subjects who are very different from their own patient population. One GP who expressed this view at its extreme called RCTs a

complete hoax because trials are done on such specific, clean questions that they never quite apply to the patient in front of you. (Project AC/PC)

Few stated it so explicitly, but a degree of scepticism was widespread, and was found across all sectors. A particularly poignant example was found by the researcher team in Project AC/PC. The hospital doctors in their study had declared RCT evidence to be largely inapplicable to their specialized practice, because they treated largely atypical patients. They claimed, therefore, that RCTs were more relevant to the run-of-the-mill patients seen in general practice. Meanwhile, in the same study, some GPs had asserted that most trials were done on very specific and carefully selected samples of patients of the sort only seen by hospital doctors and, therefore, could not readily be applied to the much less well-defined population of primary care patients. The researchers were left in this double bind wondering just where the trials did apply? If neither to consultants nor to GPs, might they be applicable among the junior hospital doctors, who saw the more routine hospital patients? The answer seemed no—or at least not directly. The juniors often told the researchers that they rarely consulted the research evidence themselves, but relied on what the consultants told them.

Broadly speaking, hospital consultants were the least sceptical about the relevance of RCTs, although Project Acute detected differences between the surgical and obstetric specialities and the other specialities. Surgeons and obstetricians were the most likely to claim that there were craft or skill elements to effective practice. GPs were more ready to doubt the relevance of trials, taking a more holistic view of other research evidence and its relevance. In general, nurses and AHPs were least sure of the relevance of RCTs to their work. This variation of views on the value of RCTs partly reflected the availability of relevant RCTs on the more practical aspects of primary care, nursing, and the therapies, where RCTs have been harder to perform and, therefore, less evidence of that type has been available.

Questions about the applicability of trial results to one's own patient population are, of course, well recognized within the conventional EBHC paradigm. Indeed, a key part of the training that doctors now receive in the critical appraisal of research papers is to ask whether the patients in the trial were similar to one's own patients. But the tenor of the views expressed here was more general. Our interviewees were not specifically criticizing studies they had accessed and appraised. Far from it, we had little or no sense of doctors routinely looking for relevant trials and then critically assessing their quality and applicability to the clinical question facing them. Rather, the widespread view expressed above about the lack of relevance of RCTs was, especially among GPs, more of a general tone of disillusionment—a sense that searching for the evidence was rarely going to be worth the effort.

A lot of our decisions are after all pretty arbitrary. Only a few can be evidence based. There are so many things where the evidence is either conflicting or not there. To sanctify evidence-based medicine could have us all diving into journals all the time. (Project GR, consultant)

Some justified this by claiming that the evidence was always changing and, was therefore, not very helpful.

The problem with glue ear is that the fashion changes every five minutes; it is useless being taught about glue ear because as soon as you think you have got it cracked they will change the fashion again. (Project AC/PC, GP)

Others, more commonly, pointed to the conflicts within the evidence. Such conflicts were often accepted as part of the general dearth of good evidence on relevant matters. One respondent, echoing a common view, stressed that the problem was not so much conflicting evidence as vast areas of uncertainty where such evidence existed as to leave one still needing to use a great deal of judgement.

Even where the most solid evidence was available, once clinicians attempted to go deeper into how to operationalize that evidence, it seemed to evanesce. For example, Project CSAG deliberately chose an area of care where good and widely accepted evidence (that stroke units saved lives) was apparently not being implemented throughout the health service. Yet, on closer observation, it was clear that even the concept of what was meant by a stroke unit was not agreed, and had been variously interpreted as a wide range of entities from an acute unit for immediate intensive care following a stroke to a dedicated rehabilitation unit for the post-acute phase of the illness. When implementing any such units, the clinicians and managers found almost no evidence on how best to design the key components, such as staffing levels or therapeutic programmes and procedures. Research evidence from trials or other sources was simply not available on the options for the organization of services or for such aspects of care. Yet this was the level of evidence the clinicians needed to implement organizational change.

The dearth of evidence on the more practical aspects of care was often stressed by nurses and therapists, who were aware that their practice—and indeed their profession—may be open to criticism as not being based on RCT evidence. One such interviewee (Project WNDP, nurse) claimed, however, that doctors eschewed non-RCT evidence as 'an excuse rather than an obstacle', since they underplayed such evidence when it was put forward by other professions, while using similar types of evidence in their own practice when it suited their purpose.

These data suggest that, in addition to the cognitively based, interprofessional differences in the interpretation and acceptance of credible evidence, there are also differences in the availability of RCT evidence. This led to differing responses among the professional groups. Some nurses and AHPs responded by wanting to try to improve their professions' research base along the biomedical model, lamenting the slow development of a trial-based research tradition that would set their work on the same plane as that of doctors. Nursing interviewees, in particular, regretted that research led by nurses was often dismissed as being of poor quality—with the reaction among some of them that nursing should, therefore, get better at RCT methodology, but among others that it should develop an alternative, more holistic approach to a distinctive evidence base for their profession. Often this was a pragmatic choice:

I think the success of evidence depends on the targets. For academics and clinicians you need RCTs and systematic reviews. For grass-roots level, you need observational stuff. (Project WNDP, nurse)

Others were more inclined to engage in 'paradigm wars', advocating a distinctive methodological scientific base for their particular profession. Such respondents, in other words, asserted that RCTs were simply not appropriate for their work, and that for their profession it would be better to establish and defend a more qualitative research paradigm that would yield more relevant and usable evidence.

For things like quality of life ... there isn't strong evidence. The problem was in ignoring qualitative assessment entirely. Now we know that there is more to be gained from qualitative analysis. (Project WNDP, project manager)

However, the fact that the medical profession held RCTs as the pre-eminent form of evidence in theory could lead to tensions over the source of evidence. In the medically dominated context of most health care in the National Health Service (NHS), research that did not meet the standards of the RCT could be contested or dismissed even where better evidence was not available. Recognizing this variation in perceptions about the differential acceptance of different forms of evidence, one interviewee explained:

[A]n important part of gaining consensus was being honest about the different levels of evidence.

In summary, one observes that different clinical professions and sub-professions varied in their views of the relative merits of the different kinds of evidence available, and in many of our studies there were data to suggest that clinicians sought out the evidence that confirmed their preferred options for treatment.

This section of our data has displayed a number of critical aspects of the interpretation by practitioners of scientific evidence. The robustness of 'sound' scientific evidence is frequently unclear to the individual. In the majority of cases, scientific evidence is disputed and there are differences of view concerning what is, or is not, 'proven'. This accords strongly with the idea that knowledge is fragile, politicized, and rhetorical (Blackler 1995) and that the acquisition and sharing of knowledge involves human agency (Tsoukas and Vladimirou 2001).

Our larger project base of empirical evidence illuminates the 'hierarchy of evidence' as a social phenomenon in health care, and demonstrates that not all clinical staff hold the same view of what constitutes 'credible' evidence. If we are to progress in understanding the career of EBHC initiatives, it is essential that these differences are recognized and explored, rather than subsumed, or we cannot understand behaviour in complex organizational settings such as health care. In developing this understanding, our enquiries need to extend to the basis upon which 'credibility' is established. Nonaka et al.

(2001) suggest that knowledge is a 'justified' true belief, that is, one which has been tested against known criteria. So understanding the foundations of this justification aids us in understanding behaviour. Additionally, Brown and Duguid (2001*a*) link the nature and content of knowledge to the social setting of practice, that is, evidence is used in context. They argue that only where there are common shared values and practices will knowledge be disseminated.

7.3.2 *Processes of accepting the research evidence: appraisal or trust?*

A common complaint was of being flooded with a surfeit of advice and information about practice (a grumble particularly levelled at guidelines). Many health professionals, therefore, felt that they needed to rely on others with more time and competence to interpret research papers and summarize the implications for practice, though this was not always the case. As one interviewee put it, GPs were particularly prone to wanting their evidence 'filtered through experts', believing that they themselves had neither the time nor the skills to do it adequately. Practitioners repeatedly told us in all the studies that they learn more from each other and from their seniors than from directly reading the evidence themselves. Many expressed a desire for succinct, but trusted, summaries of evidence. This was not, however, universal. Some clinicians did seem to want to see the evidence first hand, in order to be convinced. This would depend not only on the clinicians' belief in their own abilities to appraise the evidence reliably, but also the degree of trust that they had in the main protagonists in the arguments that were developing around them, and the degree to which doubt or dispute was emerging.

There was some variability in our studies when it came to ascertaining just how much health professionals learnt from reading the journals. Doubtless this will reflect a genuine spectrum, but we need to be cautious in interpreting the data. There was a tendency for interviewees to say what they felt was expected of them and, therefore, for doctors in particular to respond positively to questions about their reading habits, as this is generally regarded as an important part of professional practice. Indeed one of our studies was led to conclude that 'journals seem to be an external symbol of professional or group membership, rather than a means of knowledge transfer' (Project AC/PC). Certainly there was evidence that health professionals rarely read the journals of the disciplines they worked alongside, for example, GPs, nurses, and physiotherapists did not read each others' journals. Nevertheless, although many claimed to read the key journals of their own professions, many also admitted that they did not read them regularly. Some GPs explained that they did not read the *British Medical Journal*—and certainly not the research articles— because they did not have the critical reading skills necessary to interpret the evidence, or they recognized that as non-specialists they may rely unduly on something they read but which subsequently, unknown to them, turns out to be misleading. Thus, it was sometimes felt to be more reliable to be cautious, to wait for the experts to summarize the current state of thinking, or to await reinforcement from other quarters, than to change one's practice by relying on one's own amateur attempts to review research evidence.

I have always found it more convincing if somebody has written a review article looking at all the evidence and mentioned it there. So very often because it has been sifted out, it goes in the *BMJ* and if there are several letters destroying that paper later, I am not going to see that. I am not a full time diabetologist, so I am going to miss out on that. (Project PC, GP)

It may not be necessary even for the experts to summarize it explicitly. Sometimes clinicians hinted that there might be short cuts to gleaning hints about the appropriateness of relevance of a research finding by listening to a local consultant's recommendation.

Some of our interviewees recognized that this tendency to listen to, or watch the behaviour of, respected, trusted colleagues accorded a powerful role, especially to hospital consultants, but also to others such as practice partners with expertise in a particular clinical area. In one of the PACE projects, for example, practice in two neighbouring hospitals differed completely because the key consultant opinion leader in each had differing views. And the consultants were often aware of their potential influence.

[I]f I was wanting to change anticoagulation I would say: 'Look, here's a nice set of slides I've made up for you summarising the evidence—really the bullet points. You want overheads? Right here they are! You want a video? Here it is. If you want an opinion leader, here I am. And here's a little summary of these papers showing you the evidence. (Project Acute, hospital consultant)

Courses on how to critically appraise research evidence were mushrooming during the time of our studies, but they seemed to have little impact on the degree to which health professionals were using appraisal skills in practice. As a specialist clinician explained at interview:

Despite the fact that I had been on a course on critical appraisal—which I really enjoyed and got a lot out of—I simply assumed that we were being given the right evidence, that public health were doing good research. I simply don't have time to reread and critically appraise the papers. That's a job for public health, which is why we are complementary to each other. (Project PACE, hospital consultant)

This was an example where several members of a project team had all relied on each other to critically appraise the summaries of evidence that were presented to them, but no one had actually done so themselves.

We found a propensity for critical appraisal skills to be used selectively. Where there was a strong 'pull' to use evidence that seemed to offer the promise of improving poor services, the urge to assess its validity and applicability was less strong. In contrast, clinicians wishing to resist changes, urged by evidence that was being pushed onto them, were all too adept at critically scrutinizing, picking large holes in the evidence so that they could more readily dismiss it. A good example of this was in Project GR, where managers and clinicians agreed that a reduction was needed in the numbers of dilatation and curettage (D&C) operations; there was no dispute and the evidence was not closely scrutinized. However, in a neighbouring district, where key local players were motivated by local circumstances to argue more about the detail, and therefore scrutinize the evidence more closely, they concluded that the evidence on the indications for D&C was much harder to find in the literature than the published review had suggested. Other good examples were the furore raised by ear, nose, and throat (ENT) surgeons over the *Effective Health Care Bulletin* that questioned the usefulness of grommets for glue ear.

In short, evidence was less likely to be taken on trust and became the subject of negotiation if there were local reasons for questioning it; and when those questions were raised, the evidence could nearly always be found wanting, such that some negotiated compromise interpretation had to be found. A corollary was that evidence tended to be used most when there was a controversy about practice, and therefore tended to be most thoroughly and deeply probed precisely where the differing protagonists were trying to adduce evidence to make their points. It was, of course, usually at these points of weakness that the evidence often showed itself to be lacking in sufficient detail and rigour, and therefore to be most open to negotiation and compromise or perhaps outright dismissal.

Arguments over evidence required both sides to maintain their credibility so as to remain trusted by those whose actions they wished to influence. The overall impression from the studies was that trust in respected colleagues was a main determinant of acceptance of new evidence. This tended to be the principal way in which clinicians coped with informational complexity and overload. Project PC concluded, for example, that information 'depended for its validity on who was giving it and comments were made that unless the practitioner was someone who was respected by the recipient, then it was likely to be disregarded' (Project PC: 21). Interpersonal networks were, as we can see, crucial in fostering such respect and trust, and hence in the consequent acceptance—or not—of the 'filtered' evidence from colleagues. As we discussed in Chapter 6, these interpersonal networks were frequently uniprofessional, so that whilst they may facilitate the diffusion of information within the network, the separate networks may impede diffusion across professional boundaries. Trust has to be built up over time by social as well as professional interaction, with much reliance on indirect reputation, as well as day-to-day professional interactions and direct experience.

Doctors, in so far as they usually shaped the whole multiprofessional treatment agenda, often acted as gatekeepers for the research evidence that informed the care given by nurses and therapists. Nurses in primary care teams were frequently willing to alter their practice on the basis of advice from doctors, without checking the evidence themselves. They tended to get their information from the doctors in their practice, and had less involvement with local or regional professional groups. Professionals in the community, such as physiotherapists who were more isolated but might belong to national or regional groups, would tend to ask someone in their own profession. Where nurses sought to influence GP practice in areas they had expertise in—and sometimes they succeeded—it was not necessarily on the basis of research evidence, but experience or advice from experts in their own profession. Again the basis for all these interprofessional exchanges of up to date knowledge seemed to be the trust that one clinician had for the expertise and knowledge of another, not on explicit personal scrutiny of the research evidence.

Here these data re-emphasize the socially constructed nature of 'evidence'. Credibility is established through interchange in a social domain. Even senior clinical staff rely on colleagues they trust, to help them make judgements and decisions on evidence. This process should be acknowledged and used more beneficially.

7.3.3 *The role of tacit or experiential knowledge*

In many of our cases, there was substantial evidence that tacit knowledge and experience were persuasive forms of evidence. There appeared to be a circular relationship between research evidence and experience—they reinforced each other and became woven together. As we have already demonstrated, the nature of evidence is ambivalent. Its interpretation is socially constructed, with great emphasis placed upon local and at least partially tacit knowing, alongside formal, explicit knowledge. Clinical practice contains many judgements, much tinkering, reckoning, and tacit knowledge, which is more reminiscent of craft skills than traditional conceptions of science. It is rarely presented as a choice—experience or science—but as an awareness of the need to balance both.

For neither condition (asthma and glue-ear) did the majority of respondents spontaneously see the nationally available published guidance as providing the guiding principles. In both cases, the most frequently mentioned guiding principle was the respondents' individual approach where they spoke of their own personal checklist and set of procedures which they had built up through their own experience. (Project AC/PC)

In Project Acute, surgeons and obstetricians saw their work as containing strong components of tacit and experiential knowledge. Surgery was sometimes seen as a craft skill by the surgeons that did not readily transfer across sites or even individual practitioners, who might exhibit different results. In many instances, tacit knowledge and shared experience were seen as crucial adjuncts to evidence.

Evidence is more powerful where it chimes with experiential knowledge. To some extent, it is oversimplistic to treat evidence and experience as standing in opposition to each other. Clinical experience and the opinions of expert professionals are often seen as an additional form of evidence which stands alongside evidence from RCTs. (Project PACE)

As one GP explained:

If the local consultant uses it, and if there is an article in the *BMJ* and it's written by—it is from a British University and it's in the *BMJ*, then if the conclusion is that it is significant and it works, I don't look too hard at the statistics. (Project PC, GP)

A recurring theme throughout all the studies is a degree of tension between evidence and experience. Health care is essentially a personal and individualized service, provided to an amazingly varied array of clients. There are few other professional services with the same degree of individualized demand. So, many practitioners are acutely aware of the extent of variation in clients and are frequently personally affected by single examples of cases that have had poor outcomes. This introduces an element of doubt and scepticism in the approach of practitioners to 'standardized' research findings. It also introduces an emotional component to the assessment of evidence.

You don't practice on the basis of evidence, but on the basis of emotion. Until we address the emotional component of scientific judgements, we won't achieve change. (Project WNDP, consultant)

Therefore our data underline the interrelationship between the formal and academic forms of knowledge and the implicit and tacit forms. As we shall see in Chapter 8, in reality these sources are frequently intermixed and each individual practitioner has to integrate and make sense of all sources.

7.3.4   *Other sources of evidence*

Apart from the 'research world', there were three additional sources for evidence. These were the 'centre' (i.e. the Department of Health [DoH] or organizations such as health authorities [HAs] that were regarded as being agents of the centre); the commercial sector, especially the pharmaceutical industry; and patients and patient organizations. Other sources, such as the mass media, were rarely mentioned in our studies although they may have had some influence.

Clinicians tended to distrust guidelines from higher echelons of the NHS, especially the DoH. The suspicion was that such sources might be biased by a desire to save money—unless their conclusions were reinforced by other more trustworthy sources (including one's own belief that this was an appropriate way to manage the condition). Even then, lack of trust might affect the acceptance of evidence simply through professional pride or pique, when doctors felt that they were being told what to do by people whom they did not respect as being more knowledgeable than them. One group of GPs, for example, was found to be undermining a PACE project because they were annoyed that 'the centre' was telling them to do something that they believed they already did. But in general, information from the DoH or HA was notable not by the hostility it received, but by its lack of visibility in our discussions of sources of evidence and guidance. However, it was not always possible for clinicians to be able to articulate the influence of higher managerial authorities and initiatives, which may have remained hidden below the surface.

Project CSAG inquired into the influence of the DoH in some detail, as it was commissioned to evaluate the extent to which the central government's drive on what was then called 'clinical effectiveness' was having any impact on practice. The research team found that clinicians expressed mixed views about general departmental initiatives and documents designed to promulgate evidence-based medicine (EBM) or 'clinical effectiveness'; these were more likely to appeal to clinicians with management jobs than those without. In the main, they provided 'ammunition' for doctors and managers negotiating change with their colleagues. As one consultant commented, such documents made the issues topical, which made it much easier for him to question the evidence for his team's actions. However, there were many who disapproved of the way in which the NHS was trying to introduce the change. This was expressed at its extreme in a (very short!) interview:

One of the biggest barriers to delivering effective care is the sort of externally imposed nonsense that you are 'rabitting on about'. (Project CSAG, professor)

Where a shift towards clinical effectiveness was occurring, however, it was not possible to separate out the influence of the departmental documents on clinical effectiveness from that of the recent intensive promotion of EBM by other influential national agencies, including journals such as the *British Medical Journal*, colleges, and professional associations, which sometimes played a vital role. Our evidence of the limited penetration of departmental documents among clinicians, coupled with their comments on the relatively low priority accorded to them, suggested that such documents had mainly an indirect effect in changing the clinical culture.

Many commented on the danger of overload of centrally produced documents giving advice and information. Among doctors in particular, this view often turned to scepticism—at its worst, a view that such products were an irrelevant waste of NHS resources, but more often simply that they were too discursive.

Pharmaceutical representatives were a source of well-summarized and easily assimilated evidence and were, of course, well resourced to produce the kinds of attractive summaries that make it easier to get the message accepted. But they were rarely mentioned. Most practitioners, when asked, denied the influence of the 'reps', regarding them as not being trustworthy sources, whose summaries of information and evidence, however attractively produced, were to be treated with scepticism. It is not possible to discern from our data whether these less-trusted sources were, nevertheless, influential in bringing about changes in practice.

7.4 Concluding remarks

In this chapter, we have explored core conceptions of the nature of knowledge and evidence, as previously expressed in the health care and private sector literatures. We have argued that though there is limited crossover in these literatures, there are many common themes and much learning to derive from the comparisons. The knowledge management literature and the EBHC literature have largely not engaged with each other. As a result, the difference between 'evidence' and knowledge has rarely been explored or debated.

Our data reinforce and confirm with a large database the view put forward by other authors (Fairhurst and Huby 1998; Van de Ven et al. 1999; Ferlie et al. 2000; Dopson et al. 2002; Fitzgerald et al. 2003; Locock et al. 1999) that the adoption and diffusion of innovations is not a rationalistic process. Robust evidence is important, but not always dominant, and rarely sufficient. Crucially, we add to this research by identifying a number of key influences across different health care contexts, and we have sought to explain the social processes and influences that generate individual compliance.

The empirical data illustrate that different individuals and members of differing professional groups have finely nuanced views of what makes 'credible' evidence. There are considerable differences in the bases and logic underpinning these ideas. To understand professional behaviour within a context, one needs to take account of professional affiliations at national/regional level; at institutional level; and at practice level, through membership of a 'community of practice'. However, professional membership is only one influential factor in the health care context, and as we have illustrated in Chapter 5, to fully comprehend the nature of organizational context a range of interacting factors need to be taken into account. A multifactored analysis inevitably produces substantial combinations of influences that may occur in any given situation. This potential range of combinations partially accounts for the results of previous meta-analysis (Bero et al. 1998), which indicated that there was no single, dominant influence or group of influences that led to diffusion in any context. A critical implication from this is that there is no 'one best way'. An additional factor in this complexity and an integral part of the explanation for individual and group variations in behaviour is the way in which perceptions of the varied characteristics and priorities of a given context are incorporated into judgements. The crucial and active role of context has already been explored in greater detail in Chapter 5, but here we need to remind ourselves that these contextual cues are part of the processes of influence and judgement.

Our data raise serious questions concerning the nature of adoption decisions and prior conceptions of this as an individual decision. Within our data, adopting and utilizing an innovation in clinical practice consists of a set of social processes. 'Adoption' is best understood as a social process involving plurality of processes. For example, our data suggest that the sources of credible evidence are most frequently 'human' or human confirmed, rather than published. Human interchange is a crucial part of the process. The social affiliations and the social networks of individuals, therefore, both frame and constrain this interchange. Social affiliations are a major influence on adoption behaviour and on the acceptance or rejection of ideas. Within the health care context, this creates a considerable level of increased complexity in diffusion processes because of the 'tribal' and multiprofessional nature of the organizations.

The social processes displayed in the data extend well beyond mere information exchange. They include social exchanges that provide information and confirm the interpretation of knowledge and the significance of new knowledge against existing knowledge. They also include debate, which may change or sway an individual's opinion. Finally, we frequently noted that social exchanges had helped provide the means and the understanding to enable individuals to customize an innovation to suit local circumstances and populations of patients. Many of these social interactions occur at local level, within the practice group.

We noted in Chapter 6 that professional, social networks also have a critical cognitive dimension. It is apparent that in order to share cognitive frameworks one needs to share practice. Earlier in this chapter, in considering conceptual ideas concerning knowledge flows, we drew on the work of Brown and Duguid (2001*a*, 2002), who suggest that in order to understand where knowledge flows and where it sticks, we need to ask where and why practices are common. In the health care context, this becomes a crucial question, as many communities of practice in health care are typically uniprofessional. Where 'teams' and multiprofessional teams are operating, they frequently consist of cooperative working between members of differing professions, rather than a collaboration of equals. In attempting to understand and interpret our empirical data, we observe that the education and socialization of individuals into a particular profession creates epistemic cultures that are not shared between the professions. These often act as barriers to a common, shared understanding of new knowledge (Ferlie et al. 2005). In order to overcome these cognitive barriers, there either needs to be increased interprofessional working practices with genuine participation by all team members or forums for debate and facilitated interprofessional workshops to discuss the evidence on innovations and its significance.

There are some illustrations in the data of cognitive 'battles' of the forms and sources of credible evidence, which are partly political. Higher status is currently ascribed by many practitioners to research data produced from RCTs and to specific publications. Thus it is understandable that this power base will be defended. But these debates also have important cognitive content and meaning and the debates themselves need to be advanced. Why in this field is it so difficult to accept the argument that historically based views of 'science' might now be too limiting?

Our data illustrate that the codified and explicit forms of knowledge are not the sole sources or producers of action. In addition to the important influences derived from the context and the framing, and at times confining, influences of membership of professional groups with social and epistemic boundaries, clinical professionals also draw on their tacit knowledge. We have demonstrated that this is an important and under-researched resource. More work is needed to reconsider the role of experiential knowledge in action and to explore the processes of 'conversion' of tacit knowledge into more explicit and transferable knowledge.

In health care we have illustrated a complex interplay between the influence of explicit 'evidence'; prior experience and the tacit knowledge derived from that; social interactions, especially within the local context; and a variety of contextual forces. Thus knowledge can be described as more grounded and contextualized than evidence. In our next chapter, we explore how knowledge is shared in local contexts.

8

Knowledge in Action

Louise Fitzgerald, Sue Dopson, Ewan Ferlie, and Louise Locock

8.1 Introduction

This chapter builds on the foundations laid in Chapters 5, 6, and 7, in which we have presented and discussed our empirical material from a number of specific perspectives, namely the crucial part played by context in the diffusion of innovations; the complex and inhibiting attributes of professional boundaries; and the ways in which interpretations of evidence impact behaviour. Those chapters present an analysis of qualitative data from hospital and primary care settings, in order to shed light on why some attempts to introduce evidence-based health care (EBHC) succeeded where others faltered. These data illustrate and open up the intricacies and complexities of change in the National Health Service (NHS), and develop an analysis that includes the role of context during innovation and change; offers a diagnosis and explanation of the interactions within and between communities of practice and professional groups; and unfolds the complex nature of evidence itself. Our analysis reveals the limitations of the simplistic approaches to implementing research or introducing EBHC.

As we suggested at the end of Chapter 7, it is necessary to review these data holistically. In this chapter, we seek to draw together these, so far, separated strands of analysis and to develop a more refined and empirically based explanation of how knowledge moves into use and influences behaviour.

To maintain our strong empirical embeddedness, we shall accomplish this by building our analysis around a series of vignettes. These will enable us to exemplify how the different configurations of factors and influences produce differing outcomes. But before moving into the vignettes, we offer a brief review of the themes from the previous chapters.

1. The key role of context in understanding the context-specific nature of innovation. We suggest that context should not be seen as the backcloth to action, but as an interacting element in the diffusion processes.
2. The critical social role played by communities of practice in interpreting and translating evidence into contexts. We note that local professional groups work together in communities of practice, which are frequently uniprofessional. There are complex interactions between and across professional boundaries, both at this most local level and at the level of the whole institution (and indeed at societal level). These boundaries affect the motivations for seeking improvement and upgrading, and the way evidence and knowledge are perceived and interpreted. Our empirical data stress the need to understand the social and cognitive nature of these boundaries.
3. The complex nature of knowledge itself. It is ambiguous, uncertain, indeed dynamic over time, and interpretable. We reformulate the nature of 'adoption decisions'; that is, empirically we demonstrate that these do not solely focus on an 'accept/reject' of the innovation. The negotiated nature of adoption processes is traced out, focusing on a wide range of factors including the evidence supporting the innovation itself. Deciding to use new knowledge is a social and political process, which nearly always involves debate and reference to others' views. Hence, the choice of group with which people engage in this debate is also significant.

Knowledge in action is thus knowledge in use within a given context or situation. To convert knowledge into use thus involves processes of interpretation, social influence, negotiation, and, debate in communities of practice. Before it leads to behavioural change, the newer knowledge has to be actively related to what individuals already know, including what they know through their experience.

As an example of the detailed subthemes that our vignettes aim to demonstrate, we introduce empirical material to explore what motivates a practitioner to look for evidence. These examples illustrate the way in which context can influence and act on the selection of priorities. Context is most frequently described by research subjects as an external influence exerting pressure inwards to influence events inside the organizational boundary. In this section, we wish to draw attention to a complementary process of interaction from within the organization, in which organizational actors reach outwards, actively seeking out information from the external environment, because it aligns and supports their internal interests. In these examples, this process can involve players grasping at mediocre or poor evidence, if it suits their objectives.

The way in which people respond to new ideas or knowledge that emerges in the environment might be described as the very first step that knowledge takes in the journey into use. We justify this as a starting point for the holistic analysis of our empirical data by proposing that if practitioners are self-motivated, they are much more likely to see such knowledge as actionable knowledge.

Innovative behaviour in an organization can rarely be understood by focusing on the scientific knowledge or evidence as the sole influencing factor. Our empirical database suggests that there are always multiple factors at work.

In the remainder of this chapter, we move into the presentation of our vignettes to further illustrate the complexity of the social processes involved in achieving evidence-based change. We start with two positive cases, which demonstrate the high combination of positive factors required to enable an innovation to diffuse reasonably rapidly. Both these cases illustrate the strong array of positive factors, combined with the relative absence of inhibiting factors required to facilitate diffusion. By comparing these two positive cases, we can see how different combinations of factors lead to differing outcomes. In particular, these cases provide evidence of the critical importance of sound relationships between clinical professionals (and possibly managers?), and of active, local, credible opinion leaders with the skills to influence.

8.2 Illustrative vignettes

8.2.1 *Aspirin to prevent secondary cardiac incidents*

This example is a study of innovation as it occurs normally within the life of an organization. The example of aspirin is an 'outlier' case, which provides a particularly interesting and unusual combination of positive factors. This innovation focuses on persuading primary care practitioners to prescribe aspirin for patients for the prevention of secondary cardiac incidents. The scientific evidence for the efficacy of aspirin is robust and has been sustained over a period of time by a number of cumulative studies and by meta-analysis. Moreover, this evidence is clearly relevant and applicable to patients who are cared for in primary care. Indeed there is a large affected population of patients who could benefit and who, without treatment, have a probability of serious adverse outcomes. The treatment is not expensive, given the nature of the risk, and is therefore an appropriate response to the condition. The treatment suits patients, as it is easy to administer at home. This therefore increases the chance of patient compliance.

As a result of this combination of factors, the use of aspirin was targeted in many health authorities (HAs) as a priority. Among the four HA research sites, three had prioritized aspirin and two had conducted districtwide audits of the use of aspirin. (Audits may be seen as a system of quality assurance, which checks the percentage of patients who are receiving appropriate treatment.)

The micro case was drawn from a primary care practice with six doctors, many active in continuing professional education and local university departments. It was an 'early adopter' of this innovation and one partner had published a paper on this topic in the British Medical Journal. *There was, therefore, a local and credible champion from within primary care. After the publication of the article, a 'Chronic Care' special interest group was set up in the practice and met regularly to develop a protocol for the management of practice patients. This group included interested doctors, practice nurses, and attached staff.*

Once a protocol had been developed, a nurse-led arterial clinic was set up to monitor patients. The shift of responsibility for routine monitoring from doctor to nurse is important. The nursing group in the practice decided how the nurses should work in the new clinic. The practice now runs three nurse-led clinics a week, supported by a doctor. The patients come to the nurse for check-ups, reassurance, and encouragement to question the doctors. Doctors and nurses have access to further evidence (continuing professional education; membership of the British Hypertension Society; postgraduate study; and contacts with consultants and university staff) for updating. Continuing debate has led to periodic changes in the clinic regime, such as dosage, agreed across the practice.

Within this practice, there was also other evidence of frequent interchange between the professions. For example, there was a weekly practice meeting to which all staff—including receptionists and administrators—were invited (and they attended). This was a minuted meeting with published agendas and an opportunity to consider proposals for improvements. As one GP put it:

> *I think we are very team orientated and I think we recognize the other members of the team far more than other places do, and encourage them to develop their own skills and interests.*

Across all the practices studied, there was widespread and up-to-date knowledge— and adoption—of this innovation. All these practices are using aspirin. Behind this widespread adoption lay a combination of positive factors, including a particularly strong evidence base.

This innovation was, therefore, successful in shifting care to a multi-professional process on a widespread basis. The social boundaries between groups of doctors in different primary care practices were overcome through multiple means. The spread of evidence was actively supported by a top-down policy push from the HA. This was matched by a participative audit process and ownership by change champions within the study site. Since this innovation was contained within primary care, many of the professional staff involved shared some basic common values about community-based and holistic care. Thus the social barriers between doctors and nurses were easier to bridge. Finally, both doctors and nurses perceived that there were relevant incentives for participation, for example, increased autonomy and status for the nurses. In the case study site, doctors and nurses agreed role redefinition, drawing on established systems for interprofessional dialogue. It was evident that the doctors and nurses shared at least some cognitive frameworks for judging the validity and robustness of an innovation; for example, they held shared views on the criteria of what constituted 'good' primary care, and therefore the process of change presented less of a challenge. This was supported by an open culture that valued knowledge and evidence, though this was not found to exist in all general practices. So, although the innovation had to cross two key boundaries, between different organizational settings and between doctors and nurses, this was effectively managed.

The next vignette also represents a successful case of innovation diffusion, but illustrates an alternative array of multiple cues and responses.

8.2.2 *Services for heart failure*

In this example, local health groups were invited to apply for funding and facilitation in implementing research-based evidence to improve their chosen area of clinical practice. Several of the key actors in this case study site had already pinpointed a need to improve the provision of services for patients with congestive heart failure— a very serious heart condition that affects up to 10 per cent of elderly people and is a large user of NHS resources (nationally > £360 million per year). Research evidence, combined with data about local patients, had suggested that a substantial proportion of patients were likely to be receiving inappropriate drugs. Discussions had already been taking place locally when some of the protagonists heard about the national initiative and recognized that it gave them an opportunity to obtain help in implementing this much-needed change.

Key local opinion leaders in primary care had been arguing for two main changes to improve services for people with heart failure. The first was an increase in the prescription of a new type of drug, angiotensin-converting enzyme (ACE) inhibitors, to replace inappropriate and often less effective use of the more simple established treatment with diuretics. The research for this was very clear and uncontroversial, although the team found when it looked more closely that there was little clarity about clinically important details such as the dosages required. The second suggested change was an increase in direct, open access to a specialist diagnostic procedure, echocardiography, which research had shown to improve the management and, therefore, the prognosis of patients with heart failure. These two changes were discussed hand in hand, although in fact some of the team recognized that there was actually little evidence to suggest that open-access echocardiography—their preferred option—was a more effective form of service than a booked, hospital-based outpatient service.

Local resource constraints (and perhaps some failure to engage the managers sufficiently to persuade them of the need for this service) meant that an adequate echocardiography service was not available locally. Previously, there had also been limited opportunity and resource to engage primary care teams in auditing their practice, against standards that took account of the research evidence about the use of ACE inhibitors. Moreover, neither the providers of the diagnostic services nor the general practitioners (GPs) who might make use of it were fully persuaded of the need to change how things were done.

In this case, there was no professional defensiveness about the new service that was being suggested or any argument with the research evidence showing that ACE inhibitors would be superior. Nor, interestingly, was there any significant questioning about the need for open-access echocardiography services, even though the evidence that open access was the best form of provision was slim and could have been debated easily. There were several possible contextual reasons why the case for change was accepted so readily. Firstly, the project was fronted by a group of highly respected local GPs who had good relations both with the trust cardiologists and with public health, who were also closely involved and held in relatively high regard. Having this weight of key opinion leader views behind the scheme, facilitated by their good informal networks, was a potent combination for ensuring the acceptance of the proposals that they supported. Secondly, sound clinical leadership was already well established, with good relationships between the acute and primary care sectors, and this gave a strong professional impetus to improve the service. Local consultant opinion that an open-access service was required was received positively and not questioned. Thirdly, the locality had developed, in the recent past, some enthusiasm for clinical audit in primary care, with a degree of involvement by GPs in reviewing their performance against agreed standards. It was, therefore, less difficult to persuade GPs to undertake an audit of the management of heart failure, and this showed the GPs that there was considerable room for improvement in the services for heart failure. The project was able to capitalize on this recent local tradition of audit in order to engage the GPs, and to keep them involved by ensuring that one of the main strands of the project was a continuing audit. The detailed feedback this gave them on the level of improvement in the service proved to be a useful guide and motivator. Fourthly, before the project had started, there had been frustration at the inadequacy of the available echocardiography services and, therefore, when there was an opportunity to further this cause by using the momentum of the evidence-based practice movement, all the main parties recognized a common benefit. Finally, the bid for funding provided additional resources and attracted support from the pharmaceutical companies.

No one had good reason to gainsay the scheme. Cardiologists (after some initial hesitation at the thought of giving primary care direct access) recognized that it would raise the quality and standing of their service. GPs would have access to improved facilities as well as greater control, a quicker turnaround for their patients, and possible financial advantages to their practices. The HA and trust managers would improve their reputations for 'evidence-based' improvements and raise their profile in primary care. Even the pharmaceutical industry would benefit, as they would improve the sales of the ACE inhibitors; they were, therefore, willing to sponsor several aspects of the project. With such a confluence of motivations, it was hardly surprising that the evidence was so readily accepted without debate.

By itself, this congruence, mainly at the top of the organization, might not have been enough to spread the new practice among the rank-and-file clinicians. Crucially, the team from the public health department was experienced, had the backing of their executives, had good local networks among clinicians who respected their views, and was quick to co-opt the local opinion leaders in primary care and hospital cardiology. The team also had strategic thinkers and worked with and through the existing professional structures. There were many alternatives that they might have used—for example, major educational events, the development and promulgation of guidelines, or the use of the purchasing contracts as a lever for change. But they chose none of these. They recognized the crucial role of the practice managers and practice nurses in gaining entrée into the very disparate primary care practices in the vicinity. So, rather than only working directly with GPs, the team used meetings with these other practice staff members to 'warm up' the practices and get them involved in educational events, so that they could spread the word through the informal *communication networks within the practices. The project team understood that the local GPs would be resistant to being coerced into joining the project, and would also resist the promulgation of guidelines on the management of heart failure. They were aware through their good informal links that there was a general fatigue and disillusionment with the plethora of guidelines on many topics from many sources. The team also recognized that this attitude, coupled with the internal communications channels within most practices, meant that there was almost no chance of reaching the GPs by sending general advice containing information about the evidence for, and benefits of, the new ways of managing heart failure. Such letters needed to be personalized and individually named to each GP, to be succinct ('bite-sized chunks'), and to be clearly identifiable as linked to this well-received project. Written communications needed to be backed up with educational sessions tailored to the ways practices worked from day to day. The project team recognized that, to have maximum persuasive effect, the education needed to be delivered by respected opinion leaders within the existing professional networks.*

It was as a result of understanding these complex circumstances that the small but skilled team from the public health department, given relatively limited time and resources, was able to make the proposals known, accepted, and implemented. By the end of the two-year project, the team was reporting substantial shifts in clinical behaviour by the GPs; acceptance of the information pack, reinforced with a well-accepted educational programme; funding (eventually) for a new echocardiogram; the establishment of new referral systems; widespread commitment to an audit of the developing service; and the direct engagement of patients through information leaflets and the local Community Health Council (CHC). It was mainly these activities that led to the health care improvements realized by the project. Although the local team was not able to provide statistically rigorous outcome measures, there was a fall in mortality from heart failure, and a substantial fall in readmissions to hospital once patients were sent back into the community to be cared for by GPs. They also had good process measures of success. All but a handful of practices were signed up to the new service and audit, and more than three quarters of the GPs were using the new referral protocols for echocardiography. The rise of around 20 per cent in the prescriptions of ACE inhibitors and a fall of one-third in the prescriptions of some diuretics (despite a continued steady increase in 'loop' diuretics) also pointed to the success of the project.

The two vignettes discussed thus far have the most positive outcomes to be found in our suite of forty-eight cases. But even within these cases, there is nothing to indicate that robust evidence alone would have effected diffusion. Indeed, in the second case, change was achieved even though the evidence for one aspect of the proposals was slim. In each of these two cases, we see a range of other positive influencers, which collectively help to reinforce the need to change behaviour. There is robust evidence *and* there is also a large-scale patient need, where outcomes can be critical. Additionally, there are, in each case, some other positive influences, such as the ease of patient compliance. Of equal importance is the absence of any inhibiting factors.

As our other vignettes will further demonstrate, the empirical data suggest that the exercise of local, skilled influence and the processes of debate are as important as robust evidence. Reflecting on these two cases, one would stress the need for *local* leadership. We also suggest that national/regional backing may be helpful and give added weight to an initiative, but that local engagement essentially requires local credibility.

We now turn to a further set of vignettes, which present examples of cases with both strong scientific evidence to support the innovation and weaker or mixed evidence, but which incorporate a range of inhibiting factors.

8.2.3 *Managing anticoagulation provision in primary care with a computer support system*

This innovation entailed an attempted shift of routine anticoagulation provision from a hospital site to local primary care practices, starting with a pilot practice. It was observed in fieldwork in the late 1990s that diffusion of the innovation remained firmly stuck at the pilot stage and that it had not spread to further local practices.

Many hospital-based cardiac departments are overstretched and run by junior doctors who provide a basic monitoring service for patients at risk of heart attacks. Hospital-based provision of monitoring also means that patients travel further for what is a relatively routine service. In the case study, one cardiologist in the local hospital was a key supporter of the innovation, to reduce the demand on hospital clinics and also to offer patients a local, high-quality service. At the level of more general health policy, the local regional health authority (RHA) was also keen to develop a set of innovations to shift routine clinical work from secondary to primary care, and was encouraging its Research and Development (R&D) Directorate to develop promising experiments.

This initiative was designed as an evidence-based intervention sponsored by the RHA R&D Directorate. A special R&D task force assessed if patients with non-rheumatic atrial fibrillation (NRAF)—a condition associated with a higher risk of stroke—could be treated differently. The plan was to delegate traditional forms of anticoagulation monitoring and control in three ways:

1. *from the traditional hospital clinic to one and then several local primary care practices;*
2. *from a system based on junior doctors to one in which a senior nurse had an enhanced role; and*
3. *from a diagnostic process provided solely by clinicians (and often junior doctors) to one supplemented by a computer-based information and advisory system.*

This failure to diffuse readily was a curious outcome because it might have been thought that this innovation would have been adopted readily. There was a strong supporting evidence base, including randomized controlled trial (RCT) evidence. It was designed from the beginning as an evidence-based intervention and supported by the Regional R&D Directorate. It had the potential to benefit a large patient group in primary care at risk of serious adverse outcomes; it was easy to administer; there was good patient compliance; and it was relatively cheap.

But the case is characterized by the presence of multiple boundaries, all of which needed to be crossed before the innovation could diffuse. These boundaries were between people and technology; between many different professional groups, and between different organizations.

The first boundary between people and technology involves achieving the acceptance of an enhanced role for technology and, in particular, the attribution of limited decision-making to a computerized system. Crossing this boundary was not particularly problematic in practice, although some doctors expressed reservations as to whether the new technology could be adequately supported by nurses.

The second boundary was between different health care organizations. Hospital consultants, primary care doctors, and health services researchers were all employed in different organizations, each with its own logic of action and set of incentives. The consultants were employed by secondary NHS Trusts, which were seeking to export more of their routine work to primary care settings in order to control high demand levels. The GPs worked for Primary Care Groups (now Trusts). They had high levels of control over their day-to-day working practices. So both primary care practitioners and organizations were likely to resist shifts of work across the primary–secondary interface, especially where compensating resources were not made available and where medicolegal responsibility remained unclear. As one GP said:

> *[I]t is something we have become particularly sensitized to, the dumping of work onto primary care without any additional resources.*

Health services researchers were more strongly represented within the RHA R&D Directorate than in NHS Trusts or primary care practices. This regional body was seeking to promote the EBHC agenda as well as the movement of work across the primary–secondary interface, sponsoring interesting experiments. However, the RHA had little direct-line managerial power—or even channels of communication—over rank-and-file clinicians and nurses.

The third boundary was between the many different professional groups involved. The range of professional stakeholders was particularly complex in this case, including hospital-based cardiologists and haematologists, their junior doctors, doctors and senior nurses in the primary care practices, and the new professional groups of computer system designers and health services researchers grouped at regional level. All had been educated and socialized in different ways. The few change champions in the case study (a hospital-based cardiologist; a regional director of R&D who had himself been a GP in the area but who was now based at a more remote regional level) could not exert persuasive power over such a range of occupational groups.

The key shifts in workload associated with the introduction of the innovation were (a) from hospital to primary care settings, and (b) from junior doctors to a new senior nurse role. However, it was observed that the senior nurse working in local primary care practices found it difficult to enact an enhanced role in practice, remaining a somewhat isolated figure. The hospital doctors were also sceptical about the nurse's ability to support the new technology.

There was also a knowledge boundary that had to be crossed, from the R&D world of abstract knowledge (RCTs; computer system design; cost effectiveness analysis) and the clinical world of local practice and interaction with real patients. To cross this boundary, researchers had to be persuasive in communicating their evidence base to professionals in both the acute sector hospital and local primary care practices.

The case study suggested that the innovation did not generally encounter strong and explicit resistance; indeed it was often seen as a sensible idea, at least in theory. Rather the problem was that of widespread indifference, the lack of energy to diffuse the innovation across different geographical settings and occupational groups. Good research evidence was not enough to lead to action, when weighed against other considerations and priorities. The innovation was competing for time and attention with more urgent issues, and found it difficult to become a top priority for action.

Anecdotal reports from key respondents in 2004 indicated that this innovation has more recently started to diffuse to more local practices. However, the diffusion pathway was much more time-consuming and complex than originally anticipated.

This case presents a prime example of an innovation that has a strong supporting knowledge base, acknowledged as robust, and where one would, therefore, anticipate that the innovation would diffuse. But it does not. The complexity of the boundaries between the professional communities of practice and the organizational sectors account for this. In Chapter 6, we have stressed in our analysis that it is not predominantly the formal issues of organizational or sectoral boundaries that create the prime difficulties, but the impediments to understanding and agreement between different professional communities, which are cognitive in nature. So here we have a case where the positive factors are balanced by negative ones, which impede the rate of diffusion.

In our next case, concerning the implementation of improvements in diabetes care, we illustrate how these cognitive boundaries can be further exacerbated by poor or disrupted relationships. Even with the active intervention of an expert project leader, these problems cannot be effectively overcome.

8.2.4 *Diabetes care*

This was an ambitious project to improve long-term care for diabetics. It had three subcomponents: setting up a register of diabetics to enable a system of annual review; setting up a screening programme for diabetic retinopathy; and developing patient education materials. This involved disseminating guidelines developed by secondary care diabetes services to GPs and practice nurses in primary care.

As with the previous case, the project illustrates some of the difficulties of working across professional and managerial boundaries, if there are not well founded and strong prior relationships to build on. In this case, there was also a history of tension between the project steering group and the funders of the project. The steering group acknowledged that their approach to project management had been weak on occasion, that they had been overambitious, and that they had not achieved as much as they would have liked to. However, they felt judged unfairly on process measures, rather than whether they had actually improved services. They also felt they were not given enough credit for genuine learning from their mistakes:

> *How far are negative learning experiences reported? The bad experiences, getting it wrong, make the more interesting stories, but they get censored out.... The culture doesn't want negative results. There are constraints when you are reporting to funders. Good news is welcome, bad news is not. The... accountability process wants good news. (Project manager)*

The gap in expectations was felt to be partly a difference between clinical and managerial cultures. The members of the steering group were virtually all practising clinicians.

The evidence base for these innovations was somewhat fluid. The evidence suggested that good control of diabetes affects outcomes; regular review is taken as a proxy for ensuring good control. But there was limited evidence to help determine what the optimum interval between reviews is, and whether annual review is the most appropriate. The project chair argued that the available evidence was 'mainly medium, there's little gold-plated evidence'. Here we see the contested nature of much evidence. However, the context in which the project existed played an active role in the translation process being studied. For example, this site had experienced major organizational turbulence over the past few years, including staff changes at senior level and tensions between managers and clinicians. It was generally agreed that the HA had been diverted by its own problems and had not given the project sufficient attention. One interviewee commented on the fact that the project was not integrated with public health and other mainstream clinical effectiveness work in the HA. There had been several recent mergers, at both hospital trust and HA level, and the three existing hospital trusts were about to merge into one. There were political tensions between trusts in what used to be two different HAs.

Opinion leadership played a key role. At consultant physician level, it was generally felt that there were strong leaders in both trusts, and there were some enthusiastic GPs. But at the same time, concerns were expressed that some other key staff had not been involved early enough. There were also concerns about the extent to which medical opinion leaders carried weight with practice nursing colleagues, whose support was crucial. There were differing views about the extent of the steering group's influence, including mixed views about the extent to which the project had engaged GP opinion leadership. As one respondent summarized it:

> We had the great and the good on our steering group, and that was right—we needed the endorsement, the patronage, the sponsorship—but there weren't always good enough links further down the chain.

A significant problem was the fact that there were widely differing opinions about the effectiveness of retinal screening in the two trusts, ranging from hostile through neutral to tacit support. As one interviewee noted: 'You don't have to be actively hostile to cause trouble—you can cause a lot of problems just by being neutral.' Hostility was significantly worse in one of the two trusts, and it was felt that mixed messages emanating from consultants in different specialities was not helpful in persuading GPs to take part.

Some interviewees identified a problem with secondary care not always adopting the evidence-based practice they were recommending to GPs. For example, one of the opinion leaders had failed to persuade his junior doctors of the need to adhere to the process for review and fill in the appropriate data sheets. By contrast, some of the acute specialists had made clear efforts to 'make sure their own practice was up to scratch'.

In addition to the range of stakeholders and their differing viewpoints, a number of boundary issues are apparent in this case. The consultant physicians agreed they could have done more to work directly with primary care, rather than working through the HA. They recognized that one of the issues in the project was to encourage and generate working across the acute care/primary care sectors boundaries. In their view, this required 'hands-on commitment' from the consultants and not just from the project manager and team.

Another critical boundary issue was between the professions, in this case both within the medical profession and between medical and nursing professions. There were differing views about the extent to which the project depended and could rely on medical leadership, given that much of the work would actually be done by practice nurses. In the end, a crucial role was played by one of the project team members who devoted many hours to visiting practices in person, gaining trust and explaining the project:

> She sat down and had cups of tea with people like clerks, receptionists, practice nurses, whose cooperation was essential. She went in early on, and she went often, and became almost like one of them.

Finally, we see praise for the commitment of the 'wonderful, talented, clever' project manager. But this praise was tempered by concerns that he could only get so far without medical authority:

> He did a really wonderful job, but he didn't have the stethoscope and the white coat you really need.

The outcomes achieved in this case were mixed. Least progress was made on patient education; retinal screening made good progress after some teething difficulties; and progress with establishing annual review was reasonably good, but was held up by software problems and some resistance within secondary care. It was generally felt that the evidence was weak for the patient education component and that this partly accounted for its lack of progress, whereas it was strongest for retinal screening, where most change had been achieved. Annual review sat somewhere in the middle.

The example in this vignette demonstrates that where there are complex and negative, conflicting interrelationships between members of different organizations and members of differing professional groups, it is a major impediment to diffusion. Robust evidence can aid diffusion in this form of difficult context, but it is not sufficient to bridge organizational and professional boundaries.

In all the vignettes presented thus far, we have illustrated that innovation processes are a complex balance of positive and negative factors. The anticoagulation and diabetes cases that we have presented are closer to the norm or average of our empirical cases than the aspirin and heart failure cases. As such, it is critically important that we seek to understand the interplay of factors that lead to these mixed results.

Cumulatively, across the data, our cases highlight that there are some critical positive factors that occur commonly, though not uniformly. Alongside the robustness of the knowledge base, these include credible, local opinion leaders and sound interprofessional relationships. In some projects, high-quality project leadership aided progress towards improvement. On the other hand, to add to the complexity, there are critical negative factors, which also occur commonly. We note that these include the lack of engagement by a key stakeholder group, complicated by the power hierarchy that can exist in health care. The boundaries between communities of practice and professions can also create major barriers to shared understanding. These barriers need active interventions if they are to be overcome. In each case, we can account for the outcomes by assessing the balance of these positive factors against the negative ones.

In our next vignette, we seek to exemplify and further extend our themes. So far, we have shown the multiple cues that will be taken into account alongside the robustness of the evidence. In this example, we see many of the factors explored in the previous four vignettes recurring. But here the configuration of factors differs again. It demonstrates how strong, positive countervailing forces may enable serious difficulties to be overcome.

8.2.5 *Maternity care: the introduction of new service delivery systems for the care of women in childbirth, as specified in the document 'Changing Childbirth'*

This case focuses on the introduction of a new service delivery system for the care of women in childbirth, as specified in 'Changing Childbirth' (DoH 1993). This policy document set out to provide more informed choice to women and a range of options for childbirth. There is a controversy about the extent to which childbirth should be medicalized: it is not an illness, but a natural condition. Midwives and some active women's pressure groups resist extensive medicalization. Against this, obstetricians argue that the safety of the mother and child should be paramount. A national Working Group was set up that had a wide range of stakeholders with an interest in childbirth, including representatives of the professions, of mothers, and of advocacy groups. The Working Group engaged in data collection and consultation before producing its policy document 'Changing Childbirth'. This document was relatively unusual in that it specified quality criteria, such as continuity of care, and set time-constrained, implementation targets. To achieve the targets set out in the policy, change implementation called for a shift in the roles of, and interactions between, two key professions: obstetricians and midwives. It depended on the use (or even introduction) of joint guidelines for risk definition and management. There were strongly held views and vested interests for both midwives and obstetricians (and mothers!). The proposed shift from obstetricians to primary care doctors and mid-wives was highly contested. One obstetrician commented:

> *I suppose the main sweeping change has been the less active participation in pregnancy care by consultant obstetricians and more active involvement by other colleagues, namely the general practitioners and midwives. I have no idea how actively involved they are, they tell me they are and since they are accountable to themselves, they are their own masters. They have not invited me to comment, so then I believe them. (Consultant obstetrician)*

Our focus case is based on the maternity unit of an acute hospital trust, located on the fringes of a large, urban conurbation. Because the unit has a high level of demand from an ethnically mixed population, it is a service that operates under pressure. Additionally, the buildings are old and suffer from the deficiencies of outdated design. For example, the unit has to operate over three floors.

The strength of the evidence base for the proposed changes was variable and debated. The standards of evidence to support the safety of midwife-led care for low-risk mothers actually increased during the period in which these changes were implemented. But at the point of implementation, many questions remained about the precise criteria for defining 'high-' and 'low-risk' mothers and the procedures to be followed should a mother move from low to higher risk. The debate over evidence was clearly complicated by two factors: the interprofessional rivalries between obstetricians and midwives and the activities of advocacy groups, some of which were condemned as 'strident'.

Within our case study site, prior to the publication of 'Changing Childbirth' in 1993, the senior midwifery managers had begun a process of building up a protocol to allow the 'low-risk' mothers to be cared for in the community. The initial driver for these changes was the very overcrowded state of the antenatal clinics and the lack of space or staff in the hospital to improve this. The publication of the policy document allowed the staff to further justify the implementation of changes.

Several substantial changes in the organization and provision of services were gradually negotiated and agreed in this unit. These changes included the initial 'booking' meeting to be done by midwives, in which mothers were categorized according to risk factors. Low-risk mothers were cared for antenatally in the community and then came into a newly reorganized midwife-led unit to give birth. Community midwives began to operate in two group practices, in order to provide continuity of care to the mothers. An assessment unit was set up, which was open 24 hours and to which mothers could come if they experienced problems. The department also continued to operate a delivery suite, staffed by obstetricians, doctors, and midwives and supported by two operating theatres for higher-risk births.

It is evident that a number of factors accounted for this progress and the improvements to the services:

1. *Obstetricians and midwives had built sound relationships, based on trust, over a period of time. Both obstetricians and midwives in the unit expressed the view that 'most of my colleagues in the department are happy to work in a multidisciplinary way'.*
2. *The relative seniority and stability of the midwifery staff reinforced the trust and led most of the medical staff to comment on the fact that they could trust the midwives' judgements.*
3. *The political and strategic skills of one of the senior midwifery managers, who actively worked to maintain relationships and sought alliances with obstetricians who wanted change and would stimulate the questioning of systems.*
4. *The unit decided to employ a research midwife to encourage and foster the understanding of research evidence. This role helped sustain change and development and acted as a bridge between the midwives and the medical staff. The role was a relatively novel venture for the unit, especially since it had to be financed within current resources. It was an important practical and symbolic representation of the unit's commitment toward the development of research-based practice across the professions, including the midwifery profession.*

This vignette is a particularly strong example of a configuration of negative factors that are nullified by countervailing factors. As in the anticoagulation case, this innovation calls for the negotiation of interprofessional boundaries. But, unlike the anticoagulation case, at the time of the initiation of these service changes, there is partially formed scientific evidence to support the efficacy of the changes. There are no financial incentives or additional resources. So this case has multiple, severely inhibiting factors and we might anticipate limited or no progress. However, in our case study site, we note that sound relationships of trust, which had developed over time, enable the staff to surmount the barriers of professional boundaries and collaborate with implement changes. This process was led by key opinion leaders in both professions, but also had broader support. Another interesting attribute of this example is the existence of a 'top-down', policy-driven change strategy. This clearly thought-out change strategy is unusual. In essence, it enabled a combination of external and internal drivers for change to be galvanized. However, for this process to be effective, it necessitates local leaders who have a good strategic understanding. Finally, this case exemplifies that negative factors *can* be overcome with analysis, dedication, and effort.

Our last vignette neatly demonstrates the nuanced understanding of the local context that is required to engage professional staff in any specific organizational setting. In addition, it raises to the fore an issue that has been touched on briefly in discussing other vignettes—the issue of power.

8.2.6　*Glue ear*

This case study concerns a project where there was a difference of opinion as to whether it had succeeded or not. Like many others in the 1990s, the project was attempting to persuade ear, nose, and throat (ENT) surgeons to implement evidence that suggested they should undertake fewer grommet insertions when treating glue ear—a very common problem following ear infections in children and which can lead to hearing loss. It therefore represents an interesting example of where innovation requires the suspension of a clinical intervention. The three main organizational protagonists in this case were the RHA; the purchaser, which was the HA acting as commissioner of health services, and was largely led in this project by the public health department; and the local body of consultant ENT surgeons. All three parties were responding to a widely publicized report, the Effective Health Care Bulletin *on glue ear, which was a summary of available research.*

The region was developing processes whereby purchasers, as part of their performance objectives, could make demands about improving local hospital care, preferably in line with current best evidence. To achieve this, the region was using both carrots and sticks. As carrots, they offered to fund pilot schemes to explore methods of changing clinical practice and used a long history of local meetings and networks in an atmosphere of joint endeavour to invoke friendly competition between purchasers. The sticks were the increasing monitoring of performance, where future financial allocations, not to mention their personal career advancement, depended partly on performing well in this exercise.

The purchaser in this case study picked a topic that would fit their local agenda with minimum effort and maximum benefit. They chose grommets because this operation was a prime example of the kind of unnecessary clinical intervention that needed to be discouraged, but also because they were concerned about their inability to curb the activities of their surgeons, and they had public health staff who were well placed to work with ENT surgeons. Having previously found that suggestions to reduce the numbers of possibly unnecessary operations led only to 'old battles in entrenched positions', the public health physicians wanted to capitalize on the availability of a new member of staff, who had enjoyed especially good relations with ENT surgeons, and for career purposes needed to complete some research. This confluence of organizational and personal motivation and skills led the purchaser to grasp the opportunity to implement research evidence, which they believed would reduce unnecessary surgery, saving costs and improving services and health outcomes.

From the purchaser's viewpoint, as they had no means of direct performance management, they needed to appeal, on the one hand, to the surgeons' pride and competitiveness in leading the way in ENT and, on the other hand, to their fear of being seen to allow a high-profile project to fail. The purchaser also needed to ensure the soundness of the evidence on which this project was based.

The surgeons' viewpoint was that they knew about the Effective Health Care Bulletin *because their peer group nationally regarded it as highly controversial and were discussing it intently. They felt they might find themselves being dictated to by poorly informed bureaucrats, and were anxious to demonstrate that the evidence being put forward was seriously misleading. The strategy was to agree to take part in the project and work alongside the local public health physician they knew and respected. They believed that by doing so they had the best chance of showing that the simplistic assumptions made by the bulletin, and thence by region and purchaser, were dangerously wrong. This would help boost their claims for continued clinical freedom.*

The place of evidence in this initiative was thus deeply embedded in several strands of the organizational context: a national/regional desire to introduce an evidence-based culture; the purchaser's initial conviction that the evidence demanded fewer grommets; the shared view that the evidence needed to be critically examined as a necessary prerequisite for persuasive, credible argument; and the surgeons' conviction that rational dialogue would result in their favour. The surgeons' standpoint was to reject the principle of blanket clinical policies, because clinical work, they claimed, required individualized judgement based on tacit knowledge that could not be codified. For the region and the purchaser, however, it was equally anathema to allow opaque decision-making rules that allowed unexplained deviations from agreed best practice. The subsequent negotiations of acceptable explicit policy partly stemmed from conflicting organizational requirements such as these, and the resulting detailed tussles made varying demands on the use of evidence.

Over several months, this initial set of conditions involved the purchaser and the surgeons in a constructive, if tense and detailed, blow-by-blow negotiation over each aspect of care. The result was a particular view of the appropriate knowledge and evidence that should inform local practice, but along the way it became clear that the available evidence did little to help the actual clinical decisions that were needed in practice. It also became clear that evidence was being used in many differing ways.

Whether certain types of evidence were regarded as relevant depended on the motives of the actors considering them, and the negotiations often saw a struggle between incompatible sets of requirements. For example, the clinicians wanted evidence on how to safely identify dangerous conditions that might be confused with, or complicate, glue ear, while the Effective Health Care Bulletin, *the Region, and the purchaser were seeking evidence that would help to limit unnecessary interventions for straightforward cases of glue ear. Evidence about costs was another example. The Region was very concerned about, and prepared to invest in, ways to reduce costs while improving quality; evidence on costs therefore mattered. But when confronted with evidence on costs, the surgeons and purchaser, who were more concerned about improving the processes of clinical care and its quality, were disinclined to pay it much attention.*

These different perspectives on the evidence depended, in part, on the targets differing parties were expected to achieve. Furthermore, because the various stake-holders were attempting to achieve different targets, they sought different forms of evidence, none of which was available from the published research, and most of which was contestable. For example, the Region, in the context of meeting corporate NHS targets, needed evidence on the impact of reduced grommets on ENT activity, which was unobtainable from hospital data. The purchaser, in the context of persuading clinicians to change their practice, wanted—but could not find—research evidence on long-term outcomes so that they could credibly persuade clinicians of the benefits of such change. Thus the potential for talking past one another and/or for falling out during such negotiations was obvious.

For these contextual reasons, both the purchaser and the surgeons wanted the negotiations to succeed, and so they sustained their difficult dialogue over several months, each manoeuvring and weaving their way towards making joint sense and producing local practice guidelines. This work exemplified the process of 'combination' of externalized tacit knowledge with explicit knowledge from research discussed in Chapter 7. From the Region's perspective, the result amounted to a collusion to reject the clear thrust of the EBHC evidence for excessive grommet insertions. From the local protagonists' point of view, the new evidence-based guidelines were a good result, representing the best way to make sense of ambiguous and conflicting evidence and to improve local practice.

All the ENT consultants were involved in the discussions, and it emerged that they had never engaged before in such collective dialogue. Thus, for the clinical teams and the local managers, one of the successes was establishing dialogue, eliciting tacit knowledge, sharing assumptions, and undertaking rigorous and systematic reflective practice in the form of a detailed audit. But, for the Region, such improvements were little compensation for a failure to reduce the numbers of grommet insertions. This became a continuing source of tension.

This case also illustrated the highly contingent way in which knowledge could leak between the research world and the clinical world. An opinion leader, impressed by the high profile given to the project by the Region's publicity, contacted the project leader. The project leader used this as an opportunity to strengthen the scientifically based report that was required for academic purposes. The project leader further capitalized on the networks and influence of the 'outsider' to access conferences and experts in the field. Had these contingent factors been absent, the research knowledge flowing into the discussions would have been much less. All these local contextual features conspired to affect the quality and quantity of research knowledge that flowed from research into clinical practice and shaped the interpretation that was eventually agreed.

After much discussion and hard work, the purchaser and the surgeons agreed to follow up work as a compromise and agreed to collect better evidence on current practice and compare it with those aspects of the management of glue ear they agreed had good research evidence. This was a far cry from the Region's view of how the project should be run. For the Region, it had become little more than a time-consuming and expensive audit of surgical practice. For the purchaser, on the other hand, it was a qualified success. It had enhanced their local standing and increased their influence with a powerful group of clinicians. From the surgeons' point of view, it was a success because the threat of being told by bureaucrats how to practice and how to interpret research evidence had been averted. Sadly, we do not know what the patients thought!

In reflecting on the analysis of this case, a number of points may be concluded. If the evidence is contestable *and* there are differences between the stakeholders, then any negotiated solution will take a long time. It can be observed that there is only one clinical professional group involved in this case, so there are fewer professional boundary factors here. Nevertheless, the surgeons' negative views of the innovation are a critical inhibiting factor. Combined with the contestability of the evidence, this negative factor alone is sufficient to ensure that this innovation does not diffuse quickly. Money is seen as an important underpinning factor that allows resources, in terms of skilled people to be accessed, to start off the initiative. But again money is not the critical factor.

As in other cases, we observe the important role played by local knowledge. We reiterate that the exercise of local, skilled influence has been a major factor and contributes to the processes of local debate.

Throughout all our vignettes, we have demonstrated the complex configuration of context, which plays an integral part in the judgements made by stakeholders of the multiple cues. Context needs to be conceptualized as multifaceted. The heart failure and diabetes cases, in particular, underline how stakeholders may reach out and use characteristics of the context to achieve their own objectives. In these cases, we see how the stakeholders make use of the targets set by higher tiers and the incentives and finance available within a given regime to implement improvements. Targets generate attention. This results in priority being given to this specific target over other, possibly more 'worthy' objectives. Incentives, such as finance, may also create new, local change objectives as stakeholders reach out, opportunistically, to procure advantage.

8.3   Concluding remarks

In this section, we seek to review the accumulated themes that have emerged from the previous empirical chapters and from the reintegration of our findings in the vignettes in this chapter. We highlight five integrative themes arising from our analysis.

8.3.1   *Multiple cues affecting the processes of innovation utilization*

Within much of the writing on EBHC, the complex processes of successful innovation are undervalued. Our large-scale database proves that there are no simple linear relationships. Moreover, context plays a critical and integral part in these processes, so there is no 'one-size-fits-all' route to success. Nor have we found evidence to support the idea that there are contexts which will 'guarantee' success.

One main conclusion from our research is that we can observe multiple cues for individuals at organizational level within any given context. Our empirical data demonstrate situations in which these multiple cues are interpreted, weighed, and negotiated both by individuals and within and between groups. Following from this, we need to rethink how managers and other stakeholders analyse complex systems and adapt to accommodate complexity as normal. Weick (1995) suggests that as organizations are interdependent systems, we should not think in terms of straight-line cause and effect—'a' influences 'b'—but of circular strands of causal loops. The patterns of the processes are more crucial to understand than the substances. From a different perspective, the early work of the Tavistock researchers (Emery and Trist 1960; Emery 1972) suggested that if we were to understand how the 'whole system' of the organization functioned, we needed to examine these complex interrelationships. The open system itself is cyclical. Applying these ideas, analytically, to real organizations produced maps of interacting influences (Warmington et al. 1977). This form of analysis allows us to accommodate multiple influences, which engage in a specific situation in a specific way.

Koppenjan and Klijn (2004) pursue similar themes, arguing that for managers to deal with complex problems and the uncertainties, which are especially evident in public sector organizations, necessitates new processes. In relation to our findings, they propose that managers need to work to advance cross-frame learning and develop processes of negotiated knowledge. They also draw attention to the selective coupling of actors and arenas in the process of 'game management'. This is described as a process of developing social learning between parties from different backgrounds by setting up new linkages between actors and arenas and engaging in interactions. These interactions, it is argued, will seldom emerge spontaneously, but will require concerted action and facilitation, and time to build and strengthen trust and gradually develop tacit rules. Our research findings illustrate that the multiple cues presented in any given context are perceived, interpreted, and enacted by the various actors. Our data both clarify and explain that professionals have differing frames of reference from each other and from management. Thus the negotiation of knowledge will need active management.

8.3.2 *Multifaceted contexts with differential power to influence*

Through the vignettes, we describe the contextual features that commonly interact to affect the diffusion of innovations in complex professional organizations. Our analysis extends and develops conceptual understanding of organizational 'context' (Child and Smith 1987; Pettigrew 1987). Firstly, we can illustrate that context is a multidimensional and multifaceted, configured phenomenon, with aspects that are both largely external to the organizational boundaries, such as health care policy targets set by the Department of Health (DoH), and aspects that are internal, such as labour turnover among senior managers in the organization. Secondly, we demonstrate that context is not a set of static variables. We observe that the dimensions of context are not isolated, but interact in complex ways leading to unintended consequences. Thus a change of Chief Executive Officer (CEO) will frequently lead to an altered perception and prioritization of government targets. Thirdly, the vignettes illustrate the role of individual and group agency. Finally, we broaden the scope of structuration theory by conceptualizing the context as 'active', because the features of the context actively interact with, and are influenced by, the perceptions and behaviour of stakeholders during the processes of adopting innovations. They do not simply form the 'backcloth' against which innovations diffuse.

To facilitate a synthesized analysis of cues and contextual factors, we identify a number of the common mechanisms by which these interactions work in organizations. For innovations to diffuse into use, certain features of the context are perceived as core participating influences:

- the availability and engagement of local, credible, and skilled opinion leaders;
- the foundation of prior relationships, especially between different clinical professional groups and between clinicians and managers;
- the historical development of the services which influence current organization;
- the structural characteristics of the location; the complexity, volume, and configuration of the various organizational components;
- the skills available; the change management and project management capacity within the stakeholder groups;
- the support of the senior management, though this may be at a distance.

A major influence on the progress of new knowledge is the way in which it is shaped by politicking, power struggles, and debates, and the existence of the informal organizational structures, within which these 'negotiations' took place. Where there had been a history of close working, between doctors and other health professionals and managers who might be affected by the decision, the increased interprofessional trust and reduced barriers made it much more likely that the evidence would be quickly implemented, especially where it informed a widely agreed need for change. Good channels of communication among communities of practice within particular professions—for example by unidisciplinary meetings or informal social networks—did much to make new knowledge less 'sticky' and, to increase its flow. Similarly cross-professional communities of practice and, to some extent, artificially created multidisciplinary meetings and groups could reduce the stickiness of knowledge flow across the professional barriers. A good deal of the transfer and uptake of knowledge into action therefore depended on the pre-existing structures, processes, and cultures that either facilitated or hindered free and frank communication about the pros and cons of the proposed innovation. Entrenched views and resistance to uptake were much more likely to make knowledge 'sticky' where trusting communication was not already established. Access to the views of opinion leaders, their position in the hierarchy of decision-making power, and the degree of cross-professional respect that they commanded were all at least as important to the uptake of new knowledge as the source or strength of the evidence, its financial impact, or the implications for organizational change.

Thus one can observe that whilst robust evidence is important, it is not a sufficient condition to effect the use of an innovation. As a consequence, scientific evidence cannot be discussed in isolation; other sources and forms of influence, such as policy priorities, financial incentives, professional interests, and patients' wishes must be taken into account. Money is important but not necessarily critical.

8.3.3　*Evidence is important, and is translated into use through social processes*

Whilst the robustness of the scientific knowledge base is clearly important in health care, 'evidence' is frequently perceived as contestable. In our empirical examples, we repeatedly found illustrations of debates concerning the evidence. Moreover, even when there was widespread agreement on the soundness of scientific evidence, the processes of decision-making for the utlilization of the evidence and the required changes to patterns of behaviour were always made as a result of social interaction.

Evidence put into use has to be seen as a social process (Lave and Wenger 1991). Crucially our work underlines the differences between diffusion processes in professionalized organizations when compared with 'average' commercial organizations. Drawing on the work of Brown and Duguid (2001*a*), we stress the negotiation of understanding across the social and cognitive boundaries, which are generated by membership of a professional group and operate in the local communities of practice in which individuals work. Our research data underline the central role of local communities of practice, which are frequently uniprofessional, as well as professional group membership, in understanding the dynamics of local situations. Contrary to the role played by professional networks as channels of innovation dissemination (Robertson et al. 1996; Wenger 1998), these local communities of practice are difficult to influence from outside. They produce strong social and cognitive boundaries, but they are key arenas in which evidence is interpreted and enacted at local level, and implications for organizational change considered.

8.3.4 *Configuration of variables*

As a consequence of the first three integrative themes, we note the variable configurations of organizational factors from one context to another. This is not to suggest that this variability is random and, therefore, there is nothing anyone can do about it. Our data suggest that there are some patterns, but there is no uniformity. The implication of this core finding is that effective, innovative behaviour will be based in a situated analysis of the factors and the design of a relevant implementation strategy.

The term 'situated analysis' is used here following Lave and Wenger (1991) to mean who is involved, what they do, what everyday life is like, how key figures conduct themselves, and how others outside the context interact with it. Thus agent, activity, and world are perceived as mutually constitutive.

8.3.5 *Complementary collective and individual processes*

As we have already observed, the processes of debate and negotiation concerning any innovation are largely collective and are social in nature. Alongside these, there coexists a set of complementary processes, where each individual reflects on 'new' information and then combines this with the already known, including tacit knowledge, derived from experience. Thus, innovative behaviour—the movement of knowledge into use—involves both collective social processes and individual reflective ones. Again, these complementary processes are especially evident in health care, where the codified and often-written scientific evidence from research findings has to be combined with the highly influential knowledge derived from experience, and in some specialities, such as surgery, derived from craft/skill-based experience.

In interpreting research findings, our thinking draws on the ideas of Nonaka and Takeuchi (1995), when they were considering knowledge creation and spread in companies. In particular, we note that they acknowledge that explicit and tacit knowledge are not totally separate, but 'mutually complementary entities' (Nonaka and Takeuchi 1995: 61). They describe knowledge conversion as a social process and use the term 'internalization' to define the process by which explicit knowledge is converted to tacit knowledge via, for example, documentation. Within our data, we recognize that through processes of reflection and debate individuals 'merge' the new knowledge with their prior experience to create a novel cohesion of knowledge. These processes of reflection and interpretation of knowledge also contain elements of the properties of 'sense-making' as defined by Weick (1995). One of these seven properties is especially relevant here. Sense-making includes a focus on and by extracted cues. Weick underlines that this process uses subtleties and interdependencies, not just major events, and embraces reasoning based on incomplete information. Drawing on these ideas, we explain the reflection and interpretation processes we observed, as influenced by extracted and even sought-out cues, which are selected in part as a result of personal motivations and in part as a result of external factors, such as the current strategic priorities of a hospital trust. So individuals are motivated to select out certain cues, to attribute meaning, to discuss and negotiate with others concerning these interpretations, and eventually may be influenced to act.

Finally, assembling the accumulated integrative themes derived from this research, we conclude that for knowledge to become actionable knowledge, the following processes are involved:

- attention to, and interpretation of, the new evidence;
- assessment, analysis, and integration of the evidence with other multiple cues;

- perceiving, selecting, and interpreting the characteristics that are configured in the local and national contexts;
- debates on the significance of the evidence, including social processes;
- assimilation of new knowledge and already-known knowledge, including tacit knowledge;
- negotiating, weighing, and influencing the power dynamics within, and external to, the organizational boundaries.

9

Conclusion: From Evidence to Actionable Knowledge?

Ewan Ferlie

9.1 Developing a social perspective on the enactment of evidence

We have developed a *social* analysis of the career of evidence-based health care (EBHC) ideas and innovations as seen in real-world health care settings. The attempted adoption of evidence-based practice nearly always leads to attempts to change day-to-day clinical work practices, often across different professional groups. The complexities of achieving the redivision of health care labour so as to promote evidence-based practice have been underestimated in the past in what has been a science-driven rather than social science-driven literature base. A scientific perspective (understandably enough) has paid more attention to the production of high-quality knowledge than its diffusion, although the diffusion theme is now emerging as a major question in its own right.

Our social analysis is based on a large set of empirical case studies. The diffusion of the evidence-based innovations tracked in these cases was generally slow, complex, and contested. This suggests severe limits to the strength of 'science push' as an adoption mechanism: good evidence, by itself, is usually not enough to lead to change in working practices. This finding also opens up the possibility that important organizational and social processes may be operating as background 'blockers'. The diffusion of evidence-based innovations in health care is no more a predictable, rational, or linear process (confirming Van de Ven et al. 1999) than other forms of complex organizational innovation. This is an entirely unsurprising conclusion in the terms of organizational research, but is novel in the world of EBHC which has only more recently engaged with organizational forms of analysis. One contribution of our work has been to help link EBHC scholarship with a traditionally separate but relevant body of academic work on organizational innovation.

One response to this gap between EBHC policy and practice has been to accept that it is an important issue which needs addressing but to label it as a 'problem of implementation'. The implementation gap can, in this perspective, be closed through a search for powerful and generic (i.e. context-free) organizational interventions—if only we could find them—which will close this gap. Practice in the health care field will then comply with the tenets of evidence-based practice. The search for interventions within this paradigm is best conducted through EBHC and Cochrane orthodox methods (Bero et al. 1998), notably trial-based studies and systematic reviews of organizational interventions designed to promote the take-up of evidence-based medicine (EBM).

Our second response has been to develop an alternative social perspective that scripts in to a much greater extent the perspectives and concerns of the field. Evidence becomes 'real' by being enacted in micro clinical settings by local actors. This emergent and bottom-up perspective is very different from the top-down, prescriptive perspective of the 'implementation-gap' model. The field here has a voice in its own right and is not just a passive object that is 'changed' through top-down interventions.

What are the key assumptions and arguments of this alternative social perspective? As we clarified in Chapter 8, adopting and utilizing an evidence-based innovation in clinical practice fundamentally depends on a set of social processes such as sensing and interpreting new evidence; integrating it with existing evidence, including tacit evidence; its reinforcement or marginalization by professional networks and communities of practice; relating the new evidence to the needs of the local context; discussing and debating the evidence with local stakeholders; taking joint decisions about its enactment; and changing practice. Successful 'adoption' of an evidence-based practice depends on all these supportive social processes operating in the background. In the absence of all or even one of them, adoption is less likely to occur. Both the social nature of these processes and the plurality of their operation require emphasis.

In addition, field level actors have their own perspectives on EBHC which have to be taken seriously. The quotes from clinicians, nurses, and others in earlier chapters reveal a wide range of views about EBHC, not always favourable! Such opinions can, of course, evolve over time, perhaps moving from early scepticism to later support. So we deliberately talk of the 'enactment' of EBHC in local clinical settings, using a less static and top-down term than top-down 'implementation' of a received guideline or policy. We should not assume that the conditions are always right to promote the rapid diffusion of evidence-based practice. In practice, local actors may or may not see a shift to evidence-based practice as an important local priority. Even though in principle desirable, such a shift may not be seen as feasible, if it disturbs local agreements and routines or is dependent on winning extra resources. Local actors may contest available evidence on power political grounds rather than because of scholarly concerns about methodological purity. They may even hold a range of different views as to what counts as high-quality and credible evidence.

9.1.1   *Key elements of the social perspective*

Within this social perspective, the search for generic interventions is seen as a less promising strategy for promoting evidence-*informed* practice (we here use a deliberately wider term than that of evidence-based practice) than increasing the ability of actors to diagnose the nature of local contexts and the supply of skilled and context-sensitive action, especially from clinical leaders, to steer these ideas forward.

Active role of context

We started with the uncontroversial observation that the response of a clinical setting to EBHC ideas depended fundamentally on the context. While there were no 'laws' about what constituted a 'receptive context' (Pettigrew et al. 1992), our large-scale comparative database enabled us to tease out a cluster of commonly found features of receptivity discussed at the end of Chapter 8. As low-level trends or tendencies were found, it was not the case that every context was completely different or that there was no capacity at all for generalization about what features were associated with a faster rate of diffusion of evidence-based practice.

These features of contextual receptivity mixed indicators of structure and process (structural features included the degree of system complexity and volume of clinical work; more processual features included the historical development of services and a foundation of good prior relationships) with some features of action (credible opinion leaders; presence of change management and project management skills; support from senior management). We will return to the features of action later.

However, we argue (see Chapters 5 and 8) for a more sophisticated and active notion of 'organizational context' than displayed in much of the existing literature. Firstly, a more sophisticated notion acknowledges that local contexts are multidimensional, multifaceted configurations of forces, some of which can be seen as external to the agency and some, more internal. Secondly, context cannot be seen as a set of static and independent variables or an ordered series of hierarchical layers (which is how it is often portrayed), but as a syndrome of forces, which interact in complex ways and lead to unintended outcomes. We gave the example in Chapter 8 of how a change in CEO may give rise to an increased prioritization of governmental top-down targets as an important aspect of context. Thirdly, context is socially perceived and enacted (so that different individuals and groups interpret their organizational context in different ways), and is actively brought into the innovation process. It is then far more than a stage on which the play proceeds: it becomes part of the play itself.

Individuals make sense of such multiple contexts by drawing on a range of cognitive and emotional judgements to create for themselves an 'integral context' that informs their action. Yet the ways in which actors construe their environment is a social act. Collectively, they make sense of their context and thereby create—or enact—their environment in such a way as to affect and shape the impact of action. They can diagnose and then use features of context in a way that helps them achieve their objectives. Such sensing and enactment of context is rarely solely an individual activity but often takes place in small groups or mixed teams through active debate and dialogue. Indeed, local groups engage in differential sensing of context that affects their perceived incentives to engage in action to promote evidence-based practice.

Skilled action

While configuration and structuration theories stress the interplay between structure and process, these influential theoretical perspectives need to absorb and acknowledge the role of human action more fully. We found in our settings that key individuals in leadership roles were able to influence and stimulate innovation pathways actively.

The vignettes in Chapter 8 provide interesting examples of the importance of effective strategic leadership in this area. The spread of evidence-based practice amongst general practitioners (GPs) in the services for heart failure project, for example, was facilitated by the presence of an influential and skilful local public health department. The department was experienced, had senior management support, had good local clinical networks, and linked up with clinical opinion leaders. It also carefully thought about and designed the GP influence strategy.

The midwifery vignette in Chapter 8 illustrates the importance of the political and strategic skills of the local director of midwifery, who actively worked to maintain good relations with clinicians and actively sought alliances with obstetricians who wanted to promote change and who were ready to question established practices.

The vignettes also make clear that social structure still matters as much as action. The Diabetes Care vignette illustrates the lack of ability of an active and lively project manager to move the project forward despite best efforts, given that he lacked a medical power base. These vignettes suggest that powerful and skilful senior leadership can make a difference in helping reshape or develop local contexts. We will return to the important policy implications about the important role of clinical leadership later in the chapter.

9.1.2 *The professionalized organization, health care professions, and their boundaries*

These innovation processes are unfolding in professionalized organizational settings, which should be seen as different from other work settings (e.g. manufacturing, routine service businesses, small or medium enterprises). The distinctive nature of the professionalized organization needs to be acknowledged (e.g. it is one of Mintzberg's [1979] key organizational archetypes in its own right).

A consistent theme across the cases is the extreme importance of the health care professions in the diffusion of evidence-based innovations in health care (much more so than other stakeholders such as managers or patient representatives, both of which appeared to be largely invisible). Health care is a multiprofessional arena, which includes at its core the elite profession of medicine and also traditionally subordinated but now developing professions, such as nursing and allied health professionals (AHPs). Professionals, particularly doctors, still have the power to impede or facilitate diffusion of new clinical work practices. They may have lost some control at the strategic level of health care organizations (Ferlie et al. 1996), but they appear in our data still to have retained more substantial control over front-line clinical work practices.

There is a wide range of professions in health care organizations. There are power issues involved in understanding relations within health care professions, as medicine has long been the dominant field. Whilst work is moving across professional boundaries, there is little evidence of the historic power of the medical profession over the other professions being diminished, even in the new arena of EBHC. At the local level, we found examples of medical groups that continue to operate with barely any reference to, or consultation with, other professions in decision-making (e.g. joint protocol formation). While medicine remains the dominant profession, however, there are limits as the other health care professions retain substantial control over their own particular turf.

The different health care professions had finely nuanced and distinctive ideas about what made evidence 'credible'. There are important differences in the bases of fundamental logic that underpin these stances. In order to understand professionals' behaviour, therefore, we need to understand their professional affiliations and experience (e.g. national colleges, regional groupings, local community of health care practice, depth of personal engagement in multidisciplinary fora). In designing effective change processes, it is important to take account of all three levels of professional influence—national, regional, and local—and to understand how these forces have acted to socialize individual professionals.

In addition, we found that the *boundaries* between the different health care professions act as important inhibitors in the spread of evidence-based knowledge and practice across professional groups. Uniprofessional mechanisms for education, post-education training, and socialization reinforce these barriers. As explained in Chapter 6, we focus attention not so much on the physical, geographical, or formal boundaries between organizations, nor on the boundaries of a single profession, but on the underpinning social and (importantly) cognitive boundaries that membership of, and socialization into, a profession creates in relation to other professions or occupations involved in innovation spread. Cognitively, different health care professions may develop distinct research cultures and styles, publishing in unidisciplinary journals, which the other professions do not read or value. These social and cognitive boundaries can come together in a mutually reinforcing manner.

We found that research evidence does not travel well, but is 'sticky' at professional boundaries. We agree with Brown and Duguid's argument (2001*a*) that social cultural accounts of knowledge flows offer a richer perspective than a focus on the nature of the knowledge itself. By shifting the analysis to the operation of 'communities of practice', they underline the link between learning and identity that is built through participation and social contact. Knowledge may diffuse within different communities of practice but stick where practice is not shared.

So, acceptance of an innovation is often discussed within a uniprofessional 'community of practice' (Brown and Duguid 1991; Wenger 1998) such as a team of orthopaedic surgeons where there are, daily, high levels of interaction and discussion of work practices. However, our notion of a professionalized 'community of practice' is different from the non-professionalized communities of practice discussed elsewhere, which appear more flexible and improvised. The clinical communities of practice we encountered display features of greater institutionalization: they are unidisciplinary; they are 'self-sealing', and isolate themselves even from neighbouring professions; and they are highly connected to formal institutions (e.g. Royal Colleges, Medical Schools). There appeared to be poor linkages even between neighbouring communities of practice in the same health care organization. Unlike Brown and Duguid (2001*a*), we did not find that geographical proximity led to effective sharing of information. We need to refocus attention on how such boundaries between the health care professions operate, as these are critical in diffusion processes and still under-researched.

9.1.3   *A knowledge management perspective?*

The knowledge management literature has developed rapidly over the last decade but so far has not been widely accessed by many writers who work on EBHC. Debates about the production and dissemination of knowledge from outside the health care sector potentially offer new perspectives and insights, which may be of use. Key texts reviewed in Chapter 7 include the study by Nonaka and Takeuchi (1995), whose well-known analysis of the distinction between explicit and tacit forms of knowledge (and note their distinctive and non-European stand on the nature of knowledge) discusses the way they come together in a knowledge creation spiral; and Boisot's exploration (1998) of the processes of codification and abstraction that help move knowledge from a local and tacit form to a cosmopolitan and abstract form. Fincham et al. (1994) argue that we also have to understand political issues of power and interest group conflict in the generation and reception of knowledge and not see it as a purely cognitive process: knowledge can be powerful and it can threaten certain interest groups, which will then be motivated to reject it.

Alerted by Nonaka and Takeuchi's concepts, we explored in Chapter 7 how respondents assessed and utilized their own tacit or experiential clinical knowledge. In the best case examples there appeared to be a circular relationship between research evidence and experience—they reinforced each other and were woven together. At other times, there was a tension between craft knowledge and formal evidence. It should be remembered that clinical practice contains an element of judgement and tacit knowledge more reminiscent of craft skills than traditional conceptions of science. It may be unwise to force a stark choice between the two modes (experience *or* science), but there may be a need to balance both, as of course some well-known EBHC proponents (Sackett et al. 1996) recognize.

We found Tsoukas and Vladimirou's discussion (2001) of the difference between 'knowledge' and 'organizational knowledge' particularly illuminating and helpful. They seek to conceptualize the links between knowledge and organizational action. As quoted in Chapter 7, they argue that 'knowledge is the individual ability to draw distinctions within a collective domain of action, based on an appreciation of context, or theory, or both'. Knowledge is here not solely a mental attribute that resides in someone's head, but involves the exercise of judgement and interaction between the individual and some potential context for action. In turn, the exercise of judgement is based on the ability of the individual to draw distinctions and on the location of the individual within a collectively generated and sustained domain of action, in other words a 'practice'. Knowledge can thus be seen as more grounded and contextual than 'evidence'.

In some of the mainstream EBHC literature, by contrast, this potentially important distinction between evidence and knowledge is not debated. We suggest that 'evidence' (Rich 1997) here can be seen in the similar category as information, that is, refined data that provide added value. The hierarchy-of-evidence model indeed arranges studies in levels of robustness according to methodologically derived indicators of validity. There is a stress on the provision of good evidence, easy access to evidence, use of critical appraisal training to enable staff to assess evidence, and a search for interventions that facilitate faster organizational diffusion. Evidence, however, is not identical to knowledge until it is applied and used. Evidence needs to be perceived as valid and robust knowledge potentially applicable to local practice before it becomes 'actionable knowledge' (a term developed in Argyris 1999). So knowledge in action is, for us, evidence that has been converted through social processes into locally accepted knowledge, which is then put into use and leads to evidence-based change in working practices.

We have had more recourse to the knowledge management literature in this study than in our previous work, for example, drawing here on the notion of professional 'communities of practice' as an important explanatory concept (although construing them as less temporary or permeable than much of the mainstream communities of practice literature). A few other writers are now exploring the relevance of the knowledge management literature in understanding knowledge transfer processes in health care organizations. Swan et al. (2002) explore the explicit attempt by management to construct a novel community of practice in a health care organization to accelerate a radical innovation process: here a community of practice was being managed actively. By contrast, the clinical communities of practice we encountered were far more organic in nature. Bate and Robert (2002) have similarly advanced an argument about the need to move from 'information' to 'knowledge' within the context of the disappointing performance of the so-called Collaboratives, which were designed to promote clinical involvement in spreading evidence-based service change. (They see the Collaboratives as information rich, but knowledge poor. This may reflect the number of reporting requirements they face, which simultaneously increases the need to produce data for higher tiers but also erodes local ability to process it creatively.)

Knowledge management may be an interesting and important research theme for EBHC over the next five years—health care appears to be an underexplored and neglected sector despite the importance of knowledge as a fundamental attribute of health care. One key question is to explore social processes of knowledge sharing, particularly at the local level. How does knowledge get shared within local communities of practice? We would observe that local clinical settings build up histories and underlying change capacity over time (as some of the positive outliers described in the vignettes in Chapter 8 reveal). Positive features include active searching for new evidence and available mechanisms to facilitate this; a tradition of dialogue, debate, and learning in the clinical group; low power distance between medical staff and other health care professionals; an ability to handle the political aspects of organizational change; skilled and sensitive clinical leadership; and the presence of bridging roles.

9.2 Some policy implications

9.2.1 *Clinical opinion leaders and clinical leadership*

Clinical opinion leaders were frequently found to play an important role in sponsoring evidence-based innovations, as one important part of the overall jigsaw for change. Legitimate authority in health care organizations will often be more sapientially and professionally based than power- and management-led. This calls for the exercise of 'soft leadership' from well-placed clinicians (Sheaff et al. 2003). Other writers talk of the need for a shift from transactional to transformational leadership styles in health care (Spurgeon and Latham 2003) to provide vision, trust, excitement, and clinical buy-in (mobilizing qualities that are as important in EBHC as in many other health policy issues).

So, in principle, clinical opinion leaders could provide effective clinical leadership for organizational change. However, more thought needs to be given to the definition and identification of clinical opinion leaders by senior management to ensure their effective engagement in leading change. We concluded that there was no evidence that managers alone could produce effective diffusion strategies and clinical buy-in. Clinical opinion leaders may be an important mechanism through which rank-and-file professionals may be persuaded to become better engaged in the adoption of evidence-based innovations.

Subjective understandings of what a clinical opinion leader is or can do vary substantially by setting. Opinion leaders could be operating with covert as well as declared objectives and agendas. They were not always as helpful as originally hoped for by EBHC advocates: they could interact with the local system in unpredicted ways. Their effect was not always positive: indeed the influence of hostile or ambivalent opinion leaders is an important and neglected area (Dopson et al. 2002). As explained in Chapter 5, we found two major categories of opinion leaders: experts and peers. Expert opinion leaders are seen as the higher authority, able to explain the evidence and respond to academic debate. They may be important in the early stages of negotiating the evidence. Peer opinion leaders, on the other hand, are individuals who have applied the innovation in their own practice and can give colleagues confidence and support. They may be more influential in the later phases of implementation.

We concluded that clinical opinion leaders needed to have and retain genuine credibility with their colleagues to be effective, for example, continuing to practice. The danger of clinicians who step too far beyond the current norms to be credible was a recurrent theme: they needed to balance innovation and acceptance as a member of the group. Clinicians who present themselves to management as opinion leaders—perhaps in order to raise their profile—but who are not in reality are also potentially counterproductive.

Dopson and Mark (2003) take an overview of current issues in leadership research in health care organizations. We know that leadership is more likely to be effective where (*a*) it is distributed throughout the organization; (*b*) issues of professional power are understood; (*c*) the complex social relationships found in health care organizations are acknowledged and discussed; (*d*) efforts are made to harness talent from all quarters; and (*e*) the contribution of different perspectives is valued and utilized. This is essentially a pluralist view of leadership in health care. The effectiveness of a collective leadership in introducing change in health care is reinforced by the research of Denis et al. (1996). Within this pluralist view, however, the power of the professional subsystem clearly remains considerable and needs to be handled explicitly, especially through clinical leaders who also retain credibility in the management domain. We conclude that the development of clinical leaders to support EBHC is a key area for policy and indeed research in the future.

9.2.2 *Moving knowledge across boundaries*

We need to consider the possible mechanisms for moving evidence and new working practices more effectively across the social and cognitive boundaries identified. In many cases, appropriate fora for identifying, debating, and sharing such knowledge are either totally lacking or at the very least poorly integrated into clinical and organizational decision-making. A foundation of well-developed professional and, even more importantly, interprofessional fora, which generate real engagement and high attendance levels (as opposed to the operation of paper machinery that is unable to engage with health care workers), was needed for the effective debate and processing of knowledge within and across the health care professions. Such foundations were built up over time, but represent critical advantages for the most promising sites.

Sometimes bridging or facilitation roles could be helpful in reducing the timescale for shared learning and changing the negative perceptions that sometimes build up between different professional groups. At the strategic level, senior management or clinical opinion leaders can play a creative role in designing richer organizational settings that display the key features of receptivity. Groups of senior managers, both clinical and general, could also model collective processes of sharing.

9.2.3   EBHC policy in the future

EBHC is now in a mature phase in its policy life cycle. While the note of high excitement apparent in the early 1990s may have faded, EBHC has not disappeared as a policy issue (although it appears lower profile politically) but has become institutionalized in an expanding number of evidence-based protocols and treatments.

Our case study data relate to the early days of the EBHC movement when more of the decisions were being taken at a local level and by clinicians. Does this now present a dated picture? Since the late 1990s, central agencies, such as the National Institute of Clinical Excellence (NICE), have increased the production of guidance nationally and have advised ministers on national decisions as to whether the introduction of new health care technologies can be seen as effective both clinically and costwise. The new National Service Frameworks (NSFs) are putting in place a nationally consistent evidence base in particularly important service sectors (e.g. cancer services, coronary heart disease, mental health). National Health Service (NHS) commissioners have increasingly been trying to secure a demonstrable shift to evidence-based practice from health care providers through the commissioning process.

What are the implications of our research for future policy-making in the field of EBHC? Firstly, it highlights the danger of trying to do too much with too little. There was a relatively small number of cases or sites in our studies where EBHC activity led to high and quick impact on practice. In many examples, the so-called evidence was contested or attacked in the field. An implication is that it may be better to stick to a smaller number of areas with outstanding evidence *and* the potential for high pay-off (improve practice radically; eliminate a very poor tail; clear health gain) and deprioritize or downgrade activity in more contestable fields.

Secondly, there is a need to build up local systems' capacity and leadership to support EBHC. If the enactment of EBHC depends on a set of underlying social processes, underlying system capability is of critical importance. This systems perspective argues for a switch of attention and investment from short-term, stand-alone, policy 'initiatives' to drive EBHC forward to a greater focus on longer-term systems development and the capacity of the system to process the issue effectively.

Thirdly, the enactment of EBHC requires a mix of scientific knowledge and change management expertise. Nearly all proposals for EBHC have implications for the redesign of clinical work, often moving it between health care professions. These issues need to be handled explicitly as part of the EBHC change process, and by skilled interventionists in organizational change (e.g. the local public health department in one vignette in Chapter 7). We know now a considerable amount about change management in health care (Iles and Sutherland 2001): it is not a new or emergent field. Those responsible for progressing EBHC in the field should ensure that they access and utilize this literature base, where they find it helpful. Change management skills can come from a variety of sources but should be built in as part of the overall strategy for the diffusion of evidence-based innovations.

9.3   Future research needs

9.3.1   *Knowledge types and their combination*

We found that codified and explicit forms of knowledge were not the sole sources of legitimate knowledge, as clinical professionals also drew on their tacit or experiential knowledge. This is an important and under-researched type of knowledge. If users and their representatives start to take on a more important role in EBHC, what kind of knowledge will they regard as legitimate? Will it also tend to be of a more experiential nature? How will such knowledge be regarded in what have been more traditional scientific arenas?

More work is needed to consider the role of such experiential knowledge in producing service change. Should it be seen as a very different form of knowledge from explicit scientific knowledge or can it be combined with explicit knowledge through a conversion mechanism to produce a knowledge spiral?

9.3.2 *Learning from the positive outliers*

How can we stimulate greater learning from the subset of positive outliers? We have vignettes of two positive outliers in Chapter 8 that illustrate how movement towards evidence-based practice depended on a set of background conditions. In the first case of a single primary care practice, supportive factors included the nature of the change issue; strong evidence; good access, availability, and interest in the evidence; an extended role for the nurse; the presence of a local clinical opinion leader; a foundation of a multidisciplinary special interest group; and regular dialogue and debate within the practice.

In the other case, the evidence was also strong and uncontested and the new services proposed were not controversial. There was good clinical ownership in primary care and evidence of cooperative working with a cardiologist. There was a strong tradition of clinical audit. Interestingly, there was evidence of an explicit spread strategy adopted by the public health department. By the end of a two-year project, the public health team were reporting substantial shifts in GP behaviour across the patch.

It would be interesting to build up more examples of positive outliers—particularly where evidence-based practice had crossed conventional professional boundaries successfully—to try to establish whether there are any trends or tendencies apparent.

9.3.3 *Some methodological issues*

What are the signs of rigour in qualitative case-study-based research? What might be the analogue (if any) of the 'hierarchy-of-evidence' model apparent in the positivistic paradigm which, although partial and contestable, at least has the merit of forcing thought about what are higher- and lower-quality studies?

This wider debate is now apparent across different branches of qualitative Health Services Research (HSR), but has strong implications for health care management research, given that so much of it (at least in the UK) is now qualitative in nature and specifically case-study-based. Our own view (see Section 4.5) is that the further use of large-scale comparative case designs has much to recommend them, in line with Yin's concept (1999) of 'replication logic' (see also Eisenhardt 1989).

A second methodological lesson is how difficult and time consuming in practice the collection, aggregation, and analysis of large-scale comparative case study data is. The first problem is to locate a set of comparable studies that can be used for overview purposes. In principle, such sets of studies are likely to be generated by a research team that has been funded for a long-term programme of activity (rather than a single project) in this area, or by like-minded research teams coming together (as happened in this case). Clearly the short-term contract workers typically employed on NHS research and development (R&D) projects are unlikely to generate this kind of data or comparative analysis.

We need to develop clearer rules of method to enable us to take an overview across different studies. Deciding on the extent to which the seven studies included in our analysis could be seen as similar or dissimilar was complex, despite the fact that the two research teams shared similar background understandings and had been working together for a long time. So, methods for taking an overview across qualitative data need to be thought about much further.

9.3.4 *Final thoughts: a social perspective on the enactment of EBHC*

The social perspective on the enactment of EBHC developed throughout the book recasts the problem of EBHC 'implementation' in a very different light from that in which it is traditionally seen in terms of field-level resistance. Well-known advocates of EBM such as Sackett et al. (1996), as quoted in Chapter 3, have always rightly stressed that external clinical evidence can inform but never replace individual clinical expertise. In other words, experiential knowledge is important and can exist alongside formal scientific knowledge. Our analysis has additionally highlighted the fundamental social processes of knowledge search, assessment, debate, and enactment within local clinical settings. We hope to have brought together the traditionally disparate knowledge management and EBHC literatures.

For the EBHC academic community, we hope that the organizational analysis developed here will be interesting and also useful. For the knowledge management academic community we have developed a focus on professional communities of practice, together with their social and cognitive boundaries, which is distinctive and, we hope, additive to the existing knowledge management communities. These two academic communities of practice surely need to enter into further dialogue if we are to be forward in the study of EBHC enactment as a social process.

References

ABBOTT, A. (1988), *The System of the Professions: An Essay on the Division of Expert Labour*. London: University of Chicago Press.

ABRAHAMSON, E. (1991), 'Managerial Fads and Fashions—The Diffusion and Rejection of Innovations', *Academy of Management Review*, 16(3): 586–612.

AINLEY, P. (1994), *Degrees of Difference*. London: Lawrence and Wishart.

ALDRICH, H. (1979), *Organizations and Environments*. Englewood Cliffs, NJ: Prenctice-Hall.

ALFORD, R. (1975), *Health Care Politics*. London: University of Chicago Press.

ALLEN, D. (2001), *The Changing Shape of Nursing Practice: The Role of Nurses in the Hospital Division of Labour*. London and New York: Routledge.

—— and HUGHES, D. (2002), *Nursing and the Division of Labour in Health Care*. Basingstoke and New York: Palgrave Macmillan.

ARGYRIS, C. (1999), 'Actionable Knowledge: Design Causality in the Service of Consequential Theory', in C. Argyris (ed.), *On Organizational Learning*, 2nd edn. Oxford: Blackwell.

—— and SCHON, D. (1996), *Organisational Learning*. London: Addison-Wesley.

ARMSTRONG, D. (2002), 'Clinical Autonomy, Individual and Collective: The Problem of Changing Doctors' Behaviour', *Social Science and Medicine*, 55(10): 1771–7.

ATUN, R. (2003), 'Doctors and Managers Need to Speak a Common Language', *British Medical Journal*, 326: 655.

BARNES, J. (ed.) (1995), *The Cambridge Companion to Aristotle*. Cambridge: Cambridge University Press.

BATE, P. and ROBERT, G. (2002), 'Knowledge Management and Communities of Practice in the Private Sector: Lessons for Modernising the NHS in England and Wales', *Public Administration*, 80(4): 643–63.

BECK, U. (1992), *Risk Society: Towards a New Modernity*. London: Sage.

BECKER, H. S. (1962), 'The Nature of a Profession', in *National Society for the Study of Education: Education for the Profession*. Chicago: University of Chicago Press.

—— GEER, B., HUGHES, E. and STRAUSS, A. (1961), *Boys in White: Student Culture in a Medical School*. Chicago: University of Chicago Press.

BELL, D. (1999), 'The Axial Age of Technology, Foreword: 1999', in *The Coming of the Post-Industrial Society*. New York: Basic Books.

BERGER, P. L. and LUCKMAN, T. (1966), *The Social Construction of Reality. A Treatise in the Sociology of Knowledge*. London: The Penguin Press.

BERLANT, J. L. (1975), *Profession and Monopoly: A Study of Medicine in the United States and Great Britain*. Berkeley: University of California Press.

BERO, L., GRILLI, R., GRIMSHAW, J., HARVEY, E., OXMAN, A., and THOMSON, M. A. on behalf of the Cochrane Effective Practice and Organisation of Care Review Group, (1998), 'Closing the Gap Between Research and Practice: An Overview of Systematic Reviews of Interventions to Promote the Implementation of Research Findings', *British Medical Journal*, 317: 465–8.

BLACK, N. (2001), 'Evidence-Based Policy: Proceed with Care', *British Medical Journal*, 323: 275–8.

BLACKLER, F. (1995), 'Knowledge, Knowledge Work and Organisations', *Organisation Studies*, 16(6): 1021–46.

—— REED, M., and WHITAKER, A. (1993), 'Editorial Introduction: Knowledge Workers and Contemporary Organizations', *Journal of Management Studies*, 30: 851–61.

BLAXTER, M. on behalf of the BSA Medical Sociology Group (1996), 'Criteria for the Evaluation of Qualitative Research', *Medical Sociology News*, 22: 68–71.

BOISOT, M. H. (1998), *Knowledge Assets: Securing Competitive Advantage in the Information Economy*. Oxford: Oxford University Press.

BOYNE, G. (2001), 'Researching the New Public Management: The Role of Quantitative Methods' in K. McLaughlin, S. Osborne, and E. Ferlie (eds), *New Public Management: Current Trends and Future Prospects*. London: Routledge, 324–38.

BRIDGES, J. (2004), 'Workforce Matters: The Implications of a New Flexible Role in Acute Health Care', Ph.D. Thesis. London: City University.

Bristol Royal Infirmary Enquiry (2001). London: The Stationery Office.

British Social Attitudes (2003), The 20th report. London: Sage.

BROCK, D., POWELL, M., and HININGS, C. R. (1999), *Restructuring the Professional Organization*. London: Routledge.

BROWN, J. S. and DUGUID, P. (1991), 'Organizational Learning and Communities of Practice: Towards a Unified View of Working, Learning and Innovation', *Organization Science*, 2: 40–55.

—— —— (2001a), 'Knowledge and Organization: A Social-practice Perspective', *Organization Science*, 12: 198–213.

—— —— (2001b), *The Social Life of Information*. Boston, MA: Harvard Business School Press.

—— —— (2002), 'Local Knowledge: Innovation in the Networked Age', *Management Learning*, 33(4): 427–37.

BUDETTI, P., DRANOVE, D., GILLIES, R., HUANG, C., HUGHERS, E., SHORTELL, S., JONES, G., RADEMAKER, A., and REYNOLDS, K. (2000), 'Assessing the Impact of TQM and Organizational Culture on Multiple Outcomes of Care for Coronary Artery Bypass Graft Surgery Patients', *Medical Care*, 38(2): 207–17.

BURRELL, G. and MORGAN, G. (1979), *Sociological Paradigms and Organizational Analysis*. London: Heinemann Educational Books.

CALAS, M. B and SMIRNICH, L. (1999), 'Past Postmodernism? Reflections and Tentative Directions', *Academy of Management Review*, 24(4): 649–71.

CALLON, M., LAREDO, P., RABEHARISOA, V., GONADR, T., and LERAY, T. (1992), 'The Management and Evaluation of Technological Programs and the Dynamics of Techno-economic Networks: The Case of the AFME', *Research Policy*, 21: 215–36.

CAMPBELL, F. A., TRAMER, M. R., CARROLL, D., REYNOLDS, D. J., MOORE, R. A., and MCQUAY, H. J. (2001), 'Are Cannabinoids an Effective and Safe Treatment in the Management of Pain? A Qualitative Systematic Review', *British Medical Journal*, 323: 13–16.

CAMPBELL, R., POUND, P., POPE, C., BRITTEN, N., PILL, R., MORGAN, M., and DONOVAN, J. (2003), 'Evaluating Meta-Ethnography: A Synthesis of Qualitative Research on Lay Experiences of Diabetes and Diabetes Care', *Social Science and Medicine*, 56(4): 671–84.

CASSEL, E. (1997), *Doctoring: The Nature of Primary Care Medicine*. New York: Oxford University Press.

CHALMERS, I., ENKIN, M., and KEIRSE, M. J. N. C. (eds) (1989), *Effective Care in Pregnancy and Childbirth*. Oxford: Oxford University Press.

—— and ALTMAN, D. G. (eds) (1995), *Systematic Reviews*. London: BMJ Publishing Group.

CHAMBERS, D. (2000), 'An Exploration of the Influences on Evidence-Based Change to Clinical Practice: A Comparative Study of UK and US Health Care Initiatives', D.Phil. Thesis. Oxford: University of Oxford.

CHILD, J. (1972), 'Organization Structure, Environment and Performance: The Role of Strategic Choice', *Sociology*, 6: 1–22.

—— (1997), 'Strategic Choice in the Analysis of Action, Structure, Organizations and Environment: Retrospect and Prospect', *Organization Studies*, 18(1): 43–76.

—— and SMITH, C. (1987), 'The Context and Process of Organizational Transformation—Cadbury-Limited in Its Sector', *Journal of Management Studies*, 24(6): 565–93.

CLEGG, S., HARDY, C., and NORD, W. (eds) (1996), *Handbook of Organizational Studies*. London: Sage.

CM 3807 (1997), *The New NHS Modern Dependable*. London: TSO.

CM 4818 (2000), *NHS Plan: A Plan for Investment. A Plan for Reform*. London: TSO.

COCHRANE, A. L. (1971), *Effectiveness and Efficiency: Random Reflections on Health Services*. Cambridge: Royal Society of Medicine Press.

COHEN, Z. (2003), 'The Single Assessment Process: An Opportunity for Collaboration or a Threat to the Profession of Occupational Therapy?' *British Journal of Occupational Therapy*, May, 66(5).

COLEMAN, J., KATZ, E., and MENZEL, H. (1966), *Medical Innovation: A Diffusion Study*. New York: Bobbs Merrill.

COULTER, A. (2002), 'After Bristol: Putting Patients First', *British Medical Journal*, 324: 648–51.

CROMPTON, R. (1990), 'Professions in the Current Context', *Work, Employment and Society*, (Special Issue), May, 146–66.

CSAG (CLINICAL STANDARDS ADVISORY GROUP) (1998), *Clinical Effectiveness*. London: Clinical Standards Advisory Group.

DAMANPOUR, F. (1991), 'Organisational Innovation: A Meta-analysis of Effects of Determinants and Moderators', *Academy of Management Journal*, 34: 555–90.

DAVIDOFF, F., HAYNES, B., SACKETT, D., and SMITH, R. (1995), 'Evidence-Based Medicine: A New Journal to Help Doctors Identify the Information They Need', *British Medical Journal*, 310: 1085–6.

DAVIES, P. (1999), 'What is Evidence-Based Education?' *British Journal of Educational Studies*, 47(2): 108–21.

—— and BORUCH, R. (2001), 'The Campbell Collaboration', *British Medical Journal*, 323: 295–96.

DAVIES, H. T. O., NUTLEY, S. M., and SMITH, P. C. (1999), 'What Works? The Role of Evidence in Public Sector Organisations', *Public Money and Management*, 19(1): 3–5.

—— —— —— (2000), *What Works? Evidence-Based Policy and Practice in Public Services*. Bristol: The Policy Press.

DAVIS, D. A., THOMSON, M. A., OXMAN, A. D., and HAYNES, R. B. (1992), 'Evidence for the Effectiveness of CME: A Review of 50 Randomized Controlled Trials', *Journal of the American Medical Association*, 268(9): 1111–17.

—— —— —— —— (1995), 'Changing Physician Performance: A Systematic Review of the Effect of Continuing Medical Education Strategies', *Journal of the American Medical Association*, 274: 700–5.

DAWSON, S., SUTHERLAND, K., DOPSON, S., MILLER, R. with LAW, S. (1998), *The Relationship between R&D and Clinical Practice in Primary and Secondary Care: Cases of Adult Asthma and Glue Ear in Children: Final Report*. Judge Institute of Management Studies, University of Cambridge and Saïd Business School, University of Oxford.

DEEKS , J., GLANVILLE, J., and SHELDON, T. (1996), 'Undertaking Systematic Reviews of Research in Effectiveness: CRD Guidelines for Those Carrying Out or Commissioning Reviews', University of York: NHSCRD. (National Health Service Centre for Reviews and Dissemination) www.york.ac.uk/inst/crd/report4

DENIS, J. L., LANGLEY, A., and CAZALE, L. (1996), 'Leadership and Strategic Change under Ambiguity', *Organization Studies*, 17: 673–99.

—— HEBERT, Y., LANGLEY, A., LOZEAU, D., and TROTTIER, L. (2002), 'Explaining Diffusion Patterns for Complex Health Care Innovations', *Health Care Management Review*, 27(3): 60–73.

DEYKIN, D. and HAINES, A. (1996), 'Promoting the Use of Research Findings', in M. Peckham and R. Smith (eds), *Scientific Basis of Health Services*. London: BMJ Publishing Group.

DIMAGGIO, P. J. and POWELL, W. W. (1983), 'The Iron Cage Revisited: Institutional Isomorphism and Collective Rationality in Organizational Fields', *American Sociological Review*, 48 (April): 147–60.

DIXON-WOODS, M., FITZPATRICK, R. and ROBERTS, K. (2001), 'Including Qualitative Research in Systematic Reviews: Opportunities and Problems', *Journal of Evaluation in Clinical Practice*, 7(2): 125–33.

DoH (Department of Health) (1993), *Changing Childbirth, Part 1: Report of the Expert Maternity Group*. London: HMSO.

—— (1998), *A First Class Service: Quality in the New NHS*. London: DoH.

—— (2001*a*), *Involving Patients and the Public in Healthcare: A Discussion Paper*. London: DoH.

—— (2001*b*), *Building a Safer NHS for Patients: Implementing an Organization with a Memory*. London: DoH.

DONALD, A. (1998), 'The Front-Line Evidence-Based Medicine Project', *NHS Executive North Thames Regional Office Research & Development*, 30th June.

DONALDSON, L. (1996), 'The Normal Science of Structural Contingency Theory', in S. Clegg, C. Hardy, and W. Nord (eds), *Handbook of Organizational Studies*. London: Sage, 57–76.

DONOVAN, J. (2003), 'Evaluating Meta-Ethnography: A Synthesis of Qualitative Research on Lay Experiences of Diabetes and Diabetes Care', *Social Science & Medicine*, 56(4): 671–84.

DOPSON, S. (1993), 'Ambiguity & Change', Ph.D. Thesis. University of Oxford.

—— (1996), 'Doctors in Management: A Challenge to Established Debates', in J. Leopold, I. Glover, and M. Hughes (eds), *Beyond Reason? The National Health Service and the Limits of Management*. Avebury: Aldershot.

DOPSON, S. (2003), 'The Potential of the Case Study Method for Organizational Analysis'. *Policy and Politics*, 31(2): 217–26.

—— and GABBAY, J. (1995), 'Evaluation of the National Initiative Getting Research into Practice and Policy'. (Oxford Region) Department of Health.

—— and MARK, A. (2003), 'Summing up', in S. Dopson and A. Mark (eds), *Leading Health Care Organisations*. Basingstoke: Palgrave Macmillan.

—— —— LOCOCK, L., and CHAMBERS, D. (1999), 'Evaluation of the PACE Programme: Final Report'. Templeton College, University of Oxford and Wessex Institute for Health Research and Development, University of Southampton.

—— FITZGERALD, L., FERLIE, E., GABBAY, J. and LOCOCK, L. (2002), 'No Magic Targets! Changing Clinical Practice to Become More Evidence-Based', *Health Care Management Review*, 27(3): 35–47.

—— LOCOCK, L., GABBAY, J., FERLIE, E., and FITZGERALD, L. (2003), 'Evidence-Based Medicine and the Implementation Gap', *Health*, Special issue, 7(3): 311–30.

EDWARDS, N., KORNAKI, M. J., and SILVERSIN, J. (2002), 'Unhappy Doctors : What Are the Causes and What Can be Done?', *BMJ*, 324: 835–8.

EISENHARDT, K. (1989), 'Building Theories from Case Research', *Academy of Management Review*, 14(4): 532–50.

ELSTON, M. A. (1991), 'The Politics of Professional Power—Medicine in a Changing Health Service', in J. Gabe, M. Calnan, and M. Bury (eds), *The Sociology of the Health Service*. London: Routledge.

ETZIONI, A. (ed.) (1969), *Semi-professions and Their Organization*. London: Free Press.

EVANS, D. and HAINES, A. (2000), *Implementing Evidence-Based Changes in Health Care*. Abingdon: Radcliffe Medical Press.

EBM (EVIDENCE-BASED MEDICINE) WORKING GROUP (1992), 'Evidence-Based Medicine: A New Approach to Teaching the Practice of Medicine', *Journal of the American Medical Association*, 268(17): 2420–5.

EMERY, F. E. (ed.) (1972), *Systems Thinking: Selected Readings*, 3rd edn. Harmondsworth: Penguin.

—— and TRIST, E. L. (1960), *Socio-technical Systems in Management Sciences Models and Techniques*. London: Pergamon.

EXWORTHY, M. and HALFORD, S. (1999), *Professionals and the New Managerialism in the Public Sector*. Buckingham: Open University Press.

FAIRHURST, K. and HUBY, G. (1998), 'From Trial Data to Practical Knowledge: Qualitative Study of How General Practitioners Have Accessed and Used Evidence about Statin Drugs in their Management of Hypercholesterolaemia', *British Medical Journal*, 317: 1130–4.

FERLIE, E. (2000), 'Organizational Research' in N. Fulop et al. (eds), *Studying the Delivery and Organization of Health Care*. London: Routledge.

—— GABBAY, J., FITZGERALD, L., LOCOCK, L., and DOPSON, S. (2001), 'Evidence-Based Medicine and Organizational Change: An Overview of some Recent Qualitative Studies', in L. Ashburner (ed.), *Organizational Behaviour and Organizational Studies in Health Care*. Basingstoke: Palgrave Macmillan.

—— (2002), 'Public Management Research and Mode 2 Knowledge Production— Some Issues of Method', Revised paper given at EGOS Conference, Barcelona. London: Imperial College Management School.

—— ASHBURNER, L., FITZGERALD, L., and PETTIGREW, A.M. (1996), *The New Public Management in Action*. Oxford: Oxford University Press.

—— FITZGERALD, L., and WOOD, M. (2000), 'Getting Evidence into Clinical Practice: An Organisational Behaviour Perspective', *Journal of Health Services Research and Policy*, 5(1): 1–7.

—— FITZGERALD, L., WOOD, M., and HAWKINS, C. (2005), 'The (non) Spread of Innovations: The Mediating Role of Professionals', *Academy of Management Journal* (forthcoming).

FINCHAM, R., FLECK, J., PROCTOR, R., SCARBROUGH, H., TIERNEY, M. and WILLIAMS, R. (1994), *Expertise and Innovation Information Technology Strategies in the Financial Services Sector*. Oxford: Oxford University Press.

FIOL, C. M. (1996), 'Squeezing Harder Doesn't Always Work: Continuing the Search for Consistency in Innovation Research', *The Academy of Management Review*, 21(4): 1012–21.

FITZGERALD, L. (1994), 'Moving Clinicians into Management: A Professional Challenge or Threat?', *Journal of Management in Medicine*, 8(6): 32–44.

—— and DUFOUR, Y. (1997), 'Clinical Management as Boundary Management: A Comparative Analysis of Canadian and U.K. Health Care Institutions', *International Journal of Public Sector Management*, 10(1/2): 5–20.

—— and FERLIE, E. (2000), 'Professionals: Back to the Future?', *Human Relations*, 53(5): 713–38.

—— and STURT, J. (1992), 'Clinicians into Management—On the Change Agenda or Not?', *Health Service Management Research*, 5(2): 137–46.

—— DOPSON, S., FERLIE, E., GABBAY, J., and LOCOCK, L. (2001), 'Producing an Overview from Qualitative Research: The Credibility of Evidence as an Issue of Knowledge Utilisation', Working Paper, De Montfort University, Leicester: Department of HRM.

—— FERLIE, E., WOOD, M., and HAWKINS, C. (2002), 'Interlocking Interactions: The Diffusion of Innovations in Health Care', *Human Relations*, 55(12): 1429–49.

—— —— and HAWKINS, C. (2003), 'Innovation in Health Care: How Does Credible Evidence Influence Professionals?', *Health and Social Care in the Community*, 11(3): 219–28.

—— HAWKINS, C., and FERLIE, E. (1999), 'Achieving Change within Primary Care: Final Report', University of Warwick: CCSC.

FLOOD, J. (1993), 'The Governance of Law: Professions in the Management of Professions', Conference paper, University of Stirling.

FLYNN, R. et al. (1996), *Markets, Hierarchies and Networks*. Buckingham: Open University Press.

FLYVBJERG, B. (2001), *Making Social Science Matter*. Cambridge: Cambridge University Press.

FRANCIS, B. and HUMPHREYS, J. (1999), 'Enrolled Nurses and the Professionalisation of Nursing: A Comparison of Nurse Education and Skill Mix in Australia and the UK, *International Journal of Nursing Studies*, 36: 127–35.

FRANCOIS, C., LEMIEUX-CHARLES, L., and McGUIRE, W., *Using Knowledge and Evidence in Healthcare: Multidisciplinary Perspectives*. UOFT Press, ED (In press).

FREIDSON, E. (1970), *Professional Dominance: The Social Structure of Medical Care*. New York: Atherton Press.

—— (1984), 'The Changing Nature of Professional Control', *Annual Review of Sociology*, 10: 1–20.

FREIDSON, E. (1986), *Professional Powers: A Study of the Institutionalization of Formal Knowledge*. London and Chicago: University of Chicago Press.

—— (1989), *Medical Work in America: Essays on Health Care*. New Haven: Yale University Press.

—— (1994), *Professionalism Reborn: Theory, Prophecy and Policy*. Cambridge: Polity Press.

—— (2001), *Professionalism, The Third Logic*. Cambridge: Polity Press.

FULOP, N., ALLEN, P., CLARKE, A., and BLACK, N., (eds) (2001), *Studying the Organization and Delivery of Health Services: Research Methods*. London: Routledge.

GARVEY, B. and WILLIAMSON, B. (2002), *Beyond Knowledge Management, Dialogue, Creativity and the Corporate Curriculum*. Harlow: Pearson Education.

GEERTZ, C. (1973), *The Interpretation of Cultures*. New York: Basic Books.

GIBBONS, M., LIMOGES, C., NOWOTNY, H., SCHWARTZMAN, S., SCOTT, P., and GIDDENS, A. (1984), *The Constitution of Society: Outline of the Theory of Structuration*. Cambridge: Polity Press.

GLASER, B. and STRAUSS, A. (1967), *The Discovery of Grounded Theory: Strategies for Qualitative Research*. Chicago: Aldine.

GMC (General Medical Council) (2003), 'A Licence to Practise & Revalidation', April.

GOFFMAN, E. (1963), *Asylums*. London: Penguin.

GOODMAN, N. (2000), 'Who will Challenge Evidence-Based Medicine?' *Clinical Risk*, 6: 224–6.

GRAY, J. A. M. (2001), *Evidence-Based Healthcare: How to Make Health Policy and Management Decisions*, 2nd edn. Edinburgh: Churchill Livingstone.

GREENHALGH, T. P., ROBERT, R., BATE, P., KYRIAKIDOU, O., McFARLANE F., and PEACOCK, R (2004), 'How to Spread Good Ideas: A Systematic Review of the Literature and Diffusion, Dissemination and Sustainability of Innovations in Health Service Delivery and Organisation', Final Report, London NHSDO Programme.

GRIMSHAW, J. M. and RUSSEL, I. T. (1993), 'Effect of Clinical Guidelines on Medical Practice: A Systematic Review of Rigorous Evaluations', *Lancet*, 342: 1317–22.

—— CAMPBELL, M., ECCLES, M., and STEEN, I. (2000), 'Experimental and Quasi-Experimental Designs for Evaluating Guideline Implementation Strategies', *Family Practice*, 17: S11–18.

—— SHIRRAN, L., THOMAS, R., MOWATT, G., FRASER, C., BERO. L., GRILLI, R., HARVEY, E., OXMAN, A., and O'BRIEN, M. (2001), 'Changing Provider Behaviour—An Overview of Systematic Reviews of Interventions', *Medical Care*, 39(8): S2, 2–45.

GROSS, P. and ROMANO, P. (2001), 'Introduction', *Medical Care*, 39(8): S2, 1.

HAINES, A. and DONALD, A. (eds) (1998), *Getting Research Findings into Practice*. London: BMJ Publishing Group.

HAMEL, G. and PRAHALAD, C. (1994), *Competing for the Future*. Boston, MA: Harvard Business School Press.

HANNAN, M. T. and FREEMAN, J. (1977), 'The Population Ecology of Organizations', *American Journal of Sociology*, 82: 929–64.

—— —— (1989), *Organizational Ecology*. Cambridge, MA: Harvard University Press.

HUNTER, D., MARWOCH, G., and POLLITT, C. (1992), *Just Managing: Power and Culture in the National Health Service*. Basingstoke: Macmillan.

HARRISON, S. (1999), 'Clinical Autonomy and Health Policy: Past and Futures', in M. Exworthy and S. Halford (eds), *Professionals and the New Managerialism in the Public Sector*. Buckingham: Open University Press.

HATCH, M. J. (1997), *Organizational Analysis*. Oxford: Oxford University Press.

HAUG, M. (1973), 'Deprofessionalisation: An Alternative Hypothesis for the Future'. *Sociological Review Monograph*, 20: 195–211.

HAYNES, B. and HAINES, A. (1998), 'Barriers and Bridges to Evidence-Based Clinical Practice', in A. Haines and A. Donald (eds), *Getting Research into Practice*. London: BMJ Publishing Group, 79–85.

HEFCE (Higher Education Funding Council for England) (2001), 'Research in Nursing and Allied Health Professions', Report of the Task Group 3 to HEFCE and the Department of Health, HEFCE.

HININGS, C. R. and GREENWOOD, R. (1988), *The Dynamics of Strategic Change*. Oxford: Basil Blackwell.

HISS, R. G., MACDONALD, R., and DAVID, W. R. (1978), 'Identification of Physician Educational Influentials in Small Community Hospitals', *Proceedings of the Seventeenth Annual Conference in Research in Medical Education*. Washington DC: AAMC, 17, 283–8.

HOFF, T. and MCCAFFREY, D. P. (1996), 'Adapting, Resisting and Negotiating: How Physicians Cope with Organizational and Economic Change', *Work and Occupations*, 23(2): 165–89.

HOGGETT, P. (1996), 'New Modes of Control in the Public Service', *Public Administration*, 74 (Spring) 9–32.

HOGWOOD, B. W. and GUNN, L. A. (1984), *Policy Analysis for the Real World*. Oxford: Oxford University Press.

HOUSE, R., ROUSSEAU, D., and THOMAS-HUNT, M. (1995), 'The Meso Paradigm', in L. L. Cummings and B. M. Staw (eds), *Research in Organizational Behaviour: An Annual Series in Analytical Essays and Critical Reviews*. Greenwich: JAI Press, 71–114.

HUNTER, D. J. (1996), 'Rationing and Evidence-Based Medicine', *Journal of Evaluation in Clinical Practice*, 2(1): 5–8.

ILES, V. and SUTHERLAND, K. (2001), *Organisational Change: A Review for Health Care Managers, Professionals and Researchers*. London: London School of Hygiene.

JELINEK, M. and SCHOONHOVEN, C. B. (eds) (1990), *The Innovation Marathon: Lessons from High Technology Firms*. Oxford: Basil Blackwell.

JOHNSON, G. (1987), *Strategic Change and the Management Process*. Oxford: Basil Blackwell.

JOHNSON, T. (1995), 'Governmentality and the Institutionalization of Expertise', in T. Johnson, G. Larkin, and M. Saks (eds), *Health Professions and the State in Europe*. London: Routledge.

KAHN, K., TER RIET, G., GLANVILLE, J., SOWDEN, A. J., and KLEIJNEN, J. (2001), 'Undertaking Systematic Reviews of Research on Effectiveness: CRD Guidelines for those Carrying out or Commissioning Reviews', *CRD Report No. 4*. York: NHS CRD.

KIMBERLY, J. (1981), 'Managerial Innovation' in W. Starbuck and P. Nystrum (eds), *Handbook of Organisational Design*, Vol. 1. New York: Oxford University Press.

KING'S FUND (1991), *Report of a Working Party on Osteopathy*. London: King's Fund Institute.

KITCHENER, M. (1999), 'All Fur Coat and no Knickers: Contemporary Organizational Change in U.K. Hospitals', in D. Brock, M. Powell, and C. R. Hinings (eds), *Restructuring the Professional Organization*. London: Routledge.

References

KITCHENER, M. and WHIPP, R. (1997), Tracks of Change in Hospitals: A Study of Quasi-Market Transformation, *International Journal of Public Sector Management*, 10(1/2): 47–62.

KLEGON, D. (1978), 'The Sociology of the Professions: An Emerging Perspective', *Sociology of Work and Occupations*, 5(3): 259–83.

KLEIN, R. (1996), 'The NHS and the New Scientism: Solution or Delusion?' *Quarterly Journal of Medicine*, 89: 85–7.

—— (2000), From evidence-based medicine to evidence-based policy? *Journal of Health Services Research and Policy*, 5(2): 65–6.

KNORR-CETINA, K. (1999), *Epistemic Cultures: How the Sciences Make Knowledge*. Cambridge, MA: Harvard University Press.

KOPPENJAN, J. and KLIJN, E. (2004), *Managing Uncertainties in Networks. A Network Approach to Problem Solving and Decision-Making*. London and New York: Routledge.

KUHN, T. S. (1962), *The Structure of Scientific Revolutions*. London: University of Chicago Press.

—— (1970), *The Structure of Scientific Revolutions*, 2nd edn. London: University of Chicago Press.

LAKATOS, I. and MUSGRAVE, A. (eds) (1970), *Criticism and the Growth of Knowledge*. Cambridge: Cambridge University Press.

LANGLEY, A. (1999), 'Strategies for Theorising From Process Data', *Academy of Management Review*, 24(4): 691–710.

LARKIN, G. (1983), *Occupational Monopoly and Modern Medicine*, London: Tavistock.

—— (1995), 'State Control and Health Professions in the U.K. Historical Perspectives', in T. Johnson, G. Larkin, and M. Saks (eds), *Health Professions and the State in Europe*. London: Routledge.

LARKIN, G. V. (1979), 'Medical Dominance and Control: Radiographers and the Division of Labour', *Social Science & Medicine*, 13A: 179–215.

LATOUR, B. (1987), *Science in Action*, Cambridge, MA: Harvard University Press.

LAVE, J. C. and WENGER, E. (1991), *Situated Learning: Legitimate Peripheral Participation*. New York: Cambridge University Press.

LEE, T. S. (1999), *Using Qualitative Methods in Organizational Research*. Thousand Oaks, CA: Sage.

LEGGE, K. (1994), *Evaluating Planned Organisational Change*. London: Academic Press.

LEMIEUX-CHARLES, L., MCGUIRE, W., and BLINDER, I. (2002), 'Building Interorganizational Knowledge for Evidence-Based Health System Change', *Health Care Management Review*, 27(3): 48–59.

LIGHT, D. (1995), 'Countervailing Powers: A Framework for Professions in Transition', in T. Johnson, G. Larkin, and M. Saks (eds), *Health Professions and the State in Europe*. London: Routledge.

LOCOCK, L. (2001), *Maps and Journeys: Redesign in the NHS, HSMC*. Birmingham: University of Birmingham.

—— CHAMBERS, D., SURENDER, R., DOPSON, S., and GABBAY, J. (1999), 'Evaluation of the Welsh Clinical Effectiveness Initiative National Demonstration Projects: Final Report', Templeton College, Oxford and the Wessex Institute for Health Research and Development, University of Southampton.

—— , DOPSON, S., CHAMBERS, D., and GABBAY, J. (2001), 'Understanding the Role of Opinion Leaders in Improving Clinical Effectiveness', *Social Science and Medicine*, 53(6): 745–57.

Lomas, J. (1993), 'Retailing Research: Increasing the Role of Evidence in Clinical Services for Childbirth', *The Milbank Quarterly*, 71(3): 439–74.

—— and Haynes, K. B. (1988), 'A Taxononomy and Critical Review of Tested Strategies for the Application of Clinical Practice Recommendations: From "Official" to "Individual" Clinical Policy', *American Journal of Preventive Medicine*, 4: 77–94.

Maguire, S. (2002), 'Discourse and Adoption of Innovations: A Study of HIV/AIDS Treatments', *Health Care Management Review*, 27(3): 74–88.

Marnoch, G. (1996), *Doctors and Management in the National Health Service*. Buckingham: Open University Press.

Mays, N. and Pope, C. (2000), 'Quality in Qualitative Research', in C. Pope and N. Mays (eds), *Qualitative Research in Health Care*, 2nd edn. London: BMJ Publishing Group, 89–101.

—— Roberts, E., and Popay, J. (2001), 'Synthesising Research Evidence', in Fulop et al., op cit, 188–220.

McKee, L., Marnoch, G., and Dinnie, N. (1997), 'Puppetmasters or Puppets? Sources of Power and Influence in Clinical Directorates', Paper presented to the British Med. Soc. Conference, York.

McKee, M. and Clarke, A. (1995), 'Guidelines, Enthusiasms, Uncertainty, and the Limits to Purchasing', *British Medical Journal*, 310: 101–4.

McKinlay, B. (1988), 'Introduction: The Changing Character of the Medical Profession', *Millbank Quarterly*, 66(2): 1–9.

McNulty, T. (2002), 'Reengineering as Knowledge Management: A Case of Change in U.K. Health Care', *Management Learning*, 33(4): 439–58.

—— and Ferlie, E. (2002), *Reengineering Health Care: The Complexities of Organizational Transformation*. Oxford: Oxford University Press.

Meek, V. L. (1988), 'Organizational Culture: Origins and Weaknesses', *Organization Studies*, 9(4): 453–73.

Melia, K. (1987), *Learning and Working: The Occupational Socialisation of Nurses*. London: Tavistock.

Merton, R. K. (1973), *The Sociology of Science*. Chicago: University of Chicago Press.

Meyer, A. D., Tsui, A. S., and Hinings, C. R. (1993), 'Configurational Approaches to Organizational Analysis', *Academy of Management Journal*, 36(6): 1175–95.

Meyer, J. and Reeves, S. (1998), 'An Evaluation of the Introduction of the Care Coordinator Role within the General and Emergency Medicine Directorate', *Royal London Hospital: Interim Project Report*. London: City University.

Miles, M. B. and Huberman, A. M. (1984), *Analysing Qualitative Data: A Source Book for New Methods*. Beverly Hills, CA: Sage.

Mintzberg, H. (1979), *The Structuring of Organisations: A Synthesis of the Research*. Englewood Cliffs, NJ: Prentice-Hall.

—— (1983), *Structures in Fives: Designing Effective Organizations*. Englewood Cliffs, NJ: Prentice-Hall.

Montgomery, K. (1990), 'A Prospective Look at the Speciality of Medical Management', *Work and Occupations*, 17(2): 178–98.

Mosteller, F. (1981), 'Innovation and Evaluation', *Science*, 211: 881–6.

Muir Gray, J. A. (1998), 'Where's the Chief Knowledge Officer?', *British Medical Journal*, 317: 832.

208   *References*

MULROW, C. D. (1994), 'Rationale for Systematic Reviews', *British Medical Journal*, 309: 597–609.

MURPHY, E., DINGWALL, R., GREATBATCH, D., PARKER, S., and WATSON, P. (1998), 'Qualitative Research Methods in Health Technology Assessment: A Review of the Literature', *University of Southampton: NCC HTA, Health Technology Assessment*, 2(16).

NAVARRO, V. (1978), *Class Struggle, the State and Medicine*. London: Martin Robertson.

—— (2001), 'Undertaking Systematic Reviews of Research on Effectiveness', 2nd edn. University of York: NHSCRD.

NOBLIT, G. W. and HARE, R. D. (1988), *Meta-Ethnography: Synthesising Qualitative Studies*. London: Sage.

NONAKA, I. and TAKEUCHI, H. (1995), *The Knowledge-Creating Company, How Japanese Companies Create the Dynamics of Innovation*. London and New York: Oxford University Press.

—— TOYAMA, R., and KONNO, N. (2000), 'SECI, Ba and Leadership: A Unified Model of Dynamic Knowledge Creation', *Long Range Planning*, 33(1): 5–34.

—— —— —— (2001), 'SECI, Ba and Leadership: A Unified Model of Dynamic Knowledge Creation', in I. Nonaka, and D. Teece (eds), *Managing Industrial Knowledge: Creation, Transfer and Utilization*. London, California and Delhi: Sage.

OAKLEY, A. (2001), *Experiments in Knowing*. Cambridge: Polity Press.

ONG, B. N. (1998), 'Evolving Perceptions of Clinical Management in Acute Hospitals in England', *British Journal of Management*, 9: 199–210.

OSBOURNE, D. and GAEBLER, T. (1992), *Reinventing Government: How the Entrepreneurial Spirit is Transforming the Public Sector*. Reading, MA: Addison-Wesley.

PARKIN, F. (1979), *Marxism and Class Theory*. New York: Columbia University Press.

PARRY, N. and PARRY, J. (1976), *The Rise of the Medical Profession*. London: Croom Helm.

PATERSON, B. L., THORNE, S. E., CANAM, C., and JILLINGS, C. (2001), 'Meta-Study of Qualitative Health Research: A Practical Guide to Meta-Analysis and Meta-Synthesis', in *Methods in Nursing Research*, Vol. 3. London: Sage.

PATTON, M. (1978), *Utilisation Focussed Evaluation*. Beverly Hills, CA: Sage.

PATTON, M. Q. (1980), *Qualitative Evaluation Methods*. Beverly Hills, CA: Sage.

PAWSON, R. (2002), 'Evidence-Based Policy: The Promise of Realist Synthesis', *Evaluation*, 8(3): 340–58.

—— TILLEY, N. (1997), *Realistic Evaluation*. London: Sage.

PETTIGREW, A. M. (1985), *The Awakening Giant: Continuity and Change in Imperial Chemical Industries*. Oxford: Basil Blackwell.

—— (1987), 'Context and Action in the Transformation of the Firm', *Journal of Management Studies*, 24(6): 649–70.

—— (1990), 'Longitudinal Field Research on Change: Theory and Practice', *Organization Science*, 1(3): 267–92.

—— (1997), 'What is Processual Management', *Scandinavian Journal of Management*, 13(4): 337–48.

—— (1998), 'Success and Failure in Corporate Transformation Initiatives', in R. D. Galliers and W. R. J. Baets (eds), *Information Technology and Organizational Transformation*. Chichester: John Wiley.

—— and FENTON, E. (2000), *The Innovating Organization*. London: Sage.

—— and McNULTY, T. (1995), 'Power and Influence in and around the Boardroom', *Human Relations*, 46(8): 845–72.

—— —— (1998), 'Sources and Uses of Power in the Boardroom', *European Journal of Work and Organizational Psychology*, 7(2): 197–214.

—— and WHIPP, R. (1991), *Managing for Competitive Success*. Oxford: Basil Blackwell.

—— BRIGNALL, T. S., HARVEY, J., and WEBB, D. (1999), 'The Determinants of Organizational Performance: A Review of the Literature', Final Report, Warwick Business School.

—— FERLIE, E., and McKEE, L. (1992), *Shaping Strategic Change: Making Change in Large Organizations: The Case of the National Health Service*. London: Sage.

POLANY, M. (1966), *The Tacit Dimension*. Garden City, NY: Doubleday.

POPAY, J., ROGERS, A., and WILLIAM, G. (1998), 'Rationale and Standards for the Systematic Review of Qualitative Literature in Health Services Research', *Qualitative Health Research*, 8: 341–51.

PORAC, J., THOMAS, H., and BADEN-FULLER, C. (1989), 'Competitive Groups as Cognitive Communities: The Case of Scottish Knitwear Manufacturers', *Journal of Management Studies*, 26: 397–416.

PRESSMAN, J. and WILDAVSKY, A. (1973), *Implementation*. Berkeley: University of California Press.

PUGH, D. (1981), 'The Aston Programme of Research: Retrospect and Prospect', in A. H. Van de Ven and W. F. Joyce (eds), *Perspectives in Organization Design and Behaviour*. New York: Wiley, 135–66.

—— (1997), 'Does Context Determine Form?' in D. Pugh (ed.), *Organization Theory: Selected Readings*. London: Penguin.

RAELIN, J. A. (1985), 'The Basis for Professional Resistance to Managerial Control', *Human Resource Management*, 24/2 (Summer): 147–75.

—— (1986), *The Clash of Cultures, Managers and Professionals*. Boston: Harvard Business School Press.

RAFFERTY, A. M. (1992), 'Nursing Policy and the Nationalization of Nursing: The Representation of "Crisis" and the "Crisis" of Representation', in J. Robinson, A. Gray, and R. Elkan (eds), *Policy Issues in Nursing*. Milton Keynes: Open University Press.

RAGIN, C. C. (2000), *Fuzzy-Set Social Science*. Chicago: University of Chicago Press.

RAVETZ, J. R. (1973), *Scientific Knowledge and its Social Problems*. New York: Oxford University Press.

REEVES, S. and FREETH, D. (2002), 'The London Training Ward: An Innovative Interprofessional Initiative', *Journal of Interprofessional Care*, 16: 41–52.

—— —— McCRORIE, P., and PERRY, D. (2002), 'It Teaches You What to Expect in Real Life': Interprofessional Learning on a Training Ward for Medical, Nursing, Occupational Therapy and Physiotherapy Students', *Medical Education*, 36: 337–44.

RICH, R. F. (1997), 'Measuring Knowledge Utilization: Processes and Outcomes: Knowledge and Policy', *The International Journal of Knowledge Transfer and Utilization*, 10(3): 11–24.

RICHARDSON, G. and MAYNARD, A. (1995), 'Fewer Doctors? More Nurses? A Review of the Knowledge Base of Doctor–Nurse Substitution', Discussion Paper 135, Centre for Health Economics, University of York.

RIGBY, M., BOYNTON, P., GREENHALGH, T., and RUSSELL, J. (2004), 'Soft Networks for Bridging the Gap Between Research and Practice: Illuminative Evaluation of CHAIN', *British Medical Journal*, 328: 174.

ROBERTSON, M, SWAN, J., and NEWELL, S. (1996), 'The Role of Networks in the Diffusion of Technological Innovation', *Journal of Management Studies*, 33: 333–59.

ROGERS, E. (1995), *The Diffusion of Innovations*, 4th edn. New York: Free Press.

ROLFE, G., JACKSON, N., GARDNER, L., JASPER, M., and GALE, A. (1999), 'Developing the Role of the Generic Health Care Support Worker: Phase 1 of an Action Research Study', *International Journal of Nursing Studies*, 36, 323–34.

RUESCHEMEYER, D. (1983), 'Professional Autonomy and the Social Control of Expertise', in R. Dingwall and P. Lewis (eds), *The Sociology of the Professions*. London: Macmillan.

SACKETT, D., ROSENBERG, W. M. C., GRAY, J. A. M., HAYNES, R. B., and RICHARDSON, W. S. (1996), 'Evidence-Based Medicine: What it is and What it isn't', *British Medical Journal*, 312: 71–2.

SAKS, M. (1983), 'Removing the Blinkers? A Critique of Recent Contributions to the Sociology of Professions', *Sociological Review*, 31: 1–21.

—— (2003), *Orthodox and Alternative Medicine, Politics, Professionalization and Health Care*. London: Continuum.

SANDALL, J. (1995), 'Choice Continuity and Control: Changing Midwifery, towards a Sociological Perspective', *Midwifery*, 11: 201–9.

—— (1997), 'Midwives Burnout and Continuity of Care', *British Medical Journal*, 5(2): 106–11.

SANDELOWSKI, M. (1997), 'Making the Best of Things: Technology in American Nursing, 1870–1940', *Nursing History Review*, 5: 3–22.

—— and BARROSO, J. (2003), 'Classifying the Findings in Qualitative Studies', *Qualitative Health Research*, 13(7): 905–23.

SCARBROUGH, H. (1995), *The Management of Expertise*. London: Macmillan.

—— (ed.) (1996), *The Management of Expertise*. London: Macmillan.

SCHRAMM, W. (1997) 'Note on Case Studies of Instructional Media Projects', *Working Paper for the Academy of Educational Development*, Washington DC, Seminar No. 4 (December).

SCOTT POOLE, M., VAN DE VEN, A., DOOLEY, K., and HOLMES, M. E (2000), *Organizational Change and Innovation Processes: Theory and Methods for Research*. Oxford: Oxford University Press.

SECRETARY OF STATE (1997), *The New NHS*. London: Department of Health.

SHEAFF, R., ROGERS, A., PICKARD, S., MARSHALL, M., CAMPBELL, S., ROLAND, M., SIBBALD, B., and HALLIWELL, S. (2003), 'Medical Leadership in English Primary Care Networks', in S. Dopson and A. Mark (eds), op cit.

SHELDON, T. A. and CHALMERS, I. (1994), 'The UK Cochrane Centre and the NHS Centre for Reviews and Dissemination: Respective Roles within the Information Systems Strategy of the NHS R&D Programme; Coordination and Principles Underlying Collaboration', *Health Economics*, 3: 201–3.

SMIRCICH, L. and STUBBART, C. (1985), 'Strategic Management in an Enacted World', *Academy of Management Review*, 10(4): 724–36.

SMITH, R. (2001), 'Why are Doctors so Unhappy?', *British Medical Journal*, 322: 1073–4.

SPURGEON, P. and LATHAM, L. (2003), 'Pursuing Clinical Governance Through Effective Leadership', in S. Dopson and A. Mark, op cit.

STAKE, R. (1995), *The Art of Case Study Research*. Thousand Oakes, CA: Sage.

STEWART, R. (1999), 'Foreword', in S. Dopson and A. L. Mark (eds), *Organizational Behaviour in Health Care: The Research Agenda*. London: Macmillan.

STRAUSS, A. and CORBIN (1990), *Basics of Qualitative Research: Grounded Theory Procedures and Techniques*. London: Sage.

SWAN, J., SCARBROUGH, H., and ROBERTSON, M. (2002), 'The Construction of Communities of Practice in the Management of Innovation', *Management Learning*, 33(4): 477–96.

THORNE, M. (2000), 'Cultural Chameleons', *British Journal of Management*, 11(4): 325–39.

TRINDER, L. and REYNOLDS, S. (2000), *Evidence-Based Practice: A Critical Appraisal*. Oxford: Blackwell Publishing.

TROW, M. (1994), *The New Production of Knowledge*. London, Sage.

TSOUKAS, H. and MYLONOPOULOS, N. (2004), 'Introduction: Knowledge Construction and Creation in Organizations', *British Journal of Management*, 15 (Special Issue).

—— VLADIMIROU, E. (2001), 'What is Organizational Knowledge?', *Journal of Management Studies*, 38(7): 973–93.

TURNER, B. (1987), *Medical Power and Social Knowledge*. London: Sage.

UKCC (United Kingdom Central Council for Nursing, Midwifery and Health Visiting) (1987), *Project 2000: The Final Proposals*. London: UKCC.

—— (1992), *The Scope of Professional Practice*. London: UKCC.

—— (1999), *A Higher Level of Practice: The UKCC's Proposals for Recognising a Higher Level of Practice within the Post-Registration Regulatory Framework*. London: UKCC.

VAN DE VEN, A. (1992), 'Suggestions for Studying Strategy Process: A Research Note', *Strategic Management Journal*, 13(S): 169–88.

—— and SHOMAKER, M. (2002), 'Commentary: The Rhetoric of Evidence-Based Medicine', *Health Care Management Review*, 27(3): 89–91.

—— POLLEY, D., GARUD, R. and VENKATARAMAN, S. (1999), *The Innovation Journey*. Oxford: Oxford University Press.

VON KROGH, G., ROOS, J., and SLOCUM, K. (1994), 'An Essay on Corporate Epistemology', *Strategic Management Journal*, 15: 53–71.

WADDINGTON, I. (1973), 'The struggle to Reform the Royal College of Physicians 1767–1771. A Sociological Analysis', *Medical History*, April, 107–26.

WALBY, S. and GREENWALL, J. with MACKAY, L. and SOOTHILL, K. (1994), *Medicine and Nursing Professions in a Changing Health Service*. London: Sage.

WARMINGTON, A., Lupton, T., and Gibbin, I. (1977), *Organizational Behaviour and Performance: An Open Systems Approach to Change*. London: Macmillan.

WEBER, M. (1978), *Economy and Society*, Vol. 2. Berkeley: University of California Press, Chapter XIV.

—— (1990), 'Legitimate Authority and Bureaucracy', in D. Pugh (ed.), *Organization Theory: Selected Readings*, 3rd edn. London: Penguin Books.

WEICK, K. E. (1969), *The Social Psychology of Organising*, Reading, MA: Addison-Wesley.

—— (1995), *Sensemaking in Organizations*. London: Sage.

—— ROBERTS, K. H. (1993), 'Collective Mind in Organizations: Heedful Interrelating on Flight Decks', *Administrative Science Quarterly*, 38(3): 357–81.

WEISBROD, B. A. (1991), 'The Health Care Quadrilemma: An Essay on Technological Change, Insurance, Quality of Care, and Cost Containment', *Journal of Economic Literature*, 29: 523–52.

WENGER, E. (1998), *Communities of Practice*. Cambridge: Cambridge University Press.

WEST, E., BARRON, D. N., DOWSETT, J., and NEWTON, J. N. (1999), 'Hierarchies and Cliques in the Social Networks of Health Care Professionals: Implications for the Design of Dissemination Strategies', *Social Science and Medicine*, 48(5): 633–46.

WHITLEY, R. (1984), *The Intellectual and Social Organization of the Sciences*. Oxford: Oxford University Press.

—— (2000), *The Intellectual and Social Organization of the Sciences*, 2nd edn. Oxford: Oxford University Press.

WICKS, D. (1998), *Nurses and Doctors at Work: Rethinking Professional Boundaries*. Buckingham: Open University Press.

WILLIAMS and GIBSON, D.V. (1990), *Technology Transfer: A Communication Perspective*. London: Sage.

WILLIAMSON, P. (1992), 'From Dissemination to Use: Management and Organisational Barriers to the Application of Health Services Research Findings', *Health Bulletin*, 50: 8–86.

WING, S. (1994), 'Limits of Epidemiology', *Medicine and Global Survival*, 1: 74–86.

WOLFE, R. A. (1994), 'Organizational Innovation: Review Critique and Suggested Research Directions', *Journal of Management Studies*, 31(3): 405–31.

WOLINSKY, F. D. (1993), 'The Professional Dominance, Deprofessionalization, Proletarianization, and Corporatization Perspectives: An Overview and Synthesis', in F. W. Hafferty and J. B. McKinley (eds), *The Changing Medical Profession*. New York: Oxford University Press.

WOOD, M., FERLIE, E., and FITZGERALD, L. (1998), *Achieving Change in Clinical Practice: Scientific, Organisational and Behavioural Processes*. University of Warwick, CCSC.

WOODWARD, J. (1965), *Industrial Organization*. Oxford: Oxford University Press.

WOOLF, S. H., GROL, R., HUTCHINSON, A., ECCLES, M., and GRIMSHAW, J. (1999), 'Clinical Guidelines: Potential Benefits, Limitations, and Harms of Clinical Guidelines', *British Medical Journal*, 318: 527–30.

WYE, L. and MCCLENAHAN, J. (2000), *Getting Better with Evidence: Experiences of Putting Evidence into Practice*. London: King's Fund.

YIN, R. (1994), *Case Study Research: Design and Methods*, 2nd edn. London: Sage.

YIN, R. (1999), 'Enhancing the Quality of Case Studies in Health Services Research', *Health Services Research*, 34(5): 1209–24.

Index

Abbott, A. 108
Abel-Smith, Brian 28
Abrahamson, E. 82
abstraction of knowledge 108, 135, 136, 188–9
ACE inhibitors, and services for heart failure 159–60, 161
action research 52
actors
  actor network theory 9
  local 10, 183, 184
  organizational actors in the NHS 100–1
  and social processes 183–4
acute health care services
  and EBHC implementation 22, 24
  see also Warwick Acute Study
adoption decisions 156
  and EBHC implementation 23, 26
  and social processes 153, 183
agency, and structure 83–4
Agency for Health Care Research and Quality 34
Agryris, C. 9
AHPs (allied health professions) 186
  licensing of 128
  RCTs and credible evidence 140, 142, 143
Allen, D. 111–12
alternative medicine
  and credible evidence 123
  and professional boundaries 107
American management studies 11, 12, 16
anticoagulation case study 163–5, 168, 171
appraisal skills, and research evidence 146–7

appropriability model of EBHC implementation 8
Argyris, C. 190
ARIF (Aggressive Research Intelligence Facility) 88
Armstrong, D. 41
aspirin case study 157–9, 168
asthma care, and professional boundaries 126, 127
Aston Group 11, 14
autonomous professional groupings, and EBHC implementation 24–5

Bate, P. 190
Bell, D. 132
Bero, L. 18
biomedical approach
  and case studies 74
  and credible evidence 143
  and the positivistic HSR paradigm 49–50
  to EBHC implementation 17, 18–19, 25, 27, 36, 38, 40, 44–5, 47
Blackler, F. 104, 108, 132, 144
Boisot, M.H. 108, 135–6, 188
Booth, Charles 28
boundaries see professional boundaries
Boyne, G. 16
British Medical Association 107
British Medical Journal 137, 146, 149, 151, 158
Brown, J.S. 128, 130, 136, 145, 153–4, 179, 188
Business Process Reengineering Change Programmes 83

United States
  American management
    studies 11, 12, 16
  evidence-based practice
    centres 34
  medical managers 114
users
  patients' expectations of
    professionals 128
  views of credible evidence 123

Van de Ven, A. 37
variables, configuration of 179
viscous knowledge 136
Vladmirou, E. 132, 135, 144, 189
Von Krogh, G. 137

Warwick Acute Study 5, 65, 69, 73
  anticoagulation provision in
    primary care 163–5, 168, 171
  and context 88–9, 90, 98–9, 101
  and credible evidence 139, 141,
    145, 149
  maternity care 169–71, 186
  and opinion leaders 94, 96, 97
  and professional boundaries 117,
    120–21, 123–5, 125
Warwick Primary Care Study 7, 65,
  73
  aspirin to prevent secondary
    cardiac incidents 157–9, 168
  and context 88, 98–9
  and credible evidence 139, 145,
    149
  and opinion leaders 94, 97

and professional boundaries 122,
  125
Weber, Max 12, 14
  neo-Weberian school of
    professional boundaries 105
Weick, K.E. 14, 82, 175, 180
Weisbord, B.A. 35
welfare policy, and research
  evidence 28
Welsh National Demonstration
  Projects *see* WNDP (Welsh
  National Demonstration
  Projects)
Wenger, E. 10
Wicks, D. 111
Williamson, B. 135, 137
Williamson, P. 40, 133
WNDP (Welsh National
  Demonstration Projects) 7,
  65–6, 69, 74
  and context 87, 88
  and credible evidence 139, 143,
    150
  and diabetes care 165–8, 168, 175,
    186
  and opinion leaders 96
  and professional boundaries 118,
    119, 120, 123, 124
Wolfe, R.A. 134
Wood, M. 68, 72, 73
Woodward, J. 80

Yin, R. 66, 196
  *Case Study Research: Design and
    Methods* 54, 55, 56

Valeral lesi Riley My Heal